JOSEPH PETERSON

Semen Retention Miracle

Secrets of Sexual Energy Transmutation for Wealth, Health, Sex and Longevity

Copyright © 2020 by Joseph Peterson

All rights reserved. No part of this publication may be reproduced, stored or transmitted in any form or by any means, electronic, mechanical, photocopying, recording, scanning, or otherwise without written permission from the publisher. It is illegal to copy this book, post it to a website, or distribute it by any other means without permission.

First edition

This book was professionally typeset on Reedsy. Find out more at reedsy.com

Contents

Foreword		iv
1	THE GATEWAY TO GREATNESS	1
2	EVERYTHING YOU NEED TO KNOW ABOUT SEMEN	11
3	ANCIENT WISDOM ON SEMEN RETENTION	24
4	WHY SEMEN RETENTION IS SO BENEFICIAL	35
5	THE SCIENCE BEHIND SEMEN RETENTION	48
6	HOW SEMEN RETENTION MAKES YOU MORE SUCCESSFUL	62
7	NOFAP AND SEMEN RETENTION	73
8	SEX WITHOUT EJACULATION	88
9	FASTING, MEDITATION, COLD SHOWERS AND MORE	104
10	ARE THERE ANY DOWNSIDES TO SEMEN RETENTION?	113
11	CALL TO ACTION	118
12	REFERENCES	121

Foreword

'The reabsorption of semen by the blood is the strongest nourishment and, perhaps more than any other factor, it prompts the stimulus of power.'
(*Friedrich Nietzsche*)

'The major reason why the majority of men who succeed do not begin to do so before the age of forty to fifty, is their tendency to dissipate their energies through over-indulgence in physical expression of the emotion of sex.'
(*Napoleon Hill*)

'Falling of semen brings death; preservation of semen gives life. Semen is the real vitality in man. It is the hidden treasure for man.'
(*The Yogaśāstra — 12th century*)

'I don't waste my essence in bed.'
(*Winston Churchill*)

1

THE GATEWAY TO GREATNESS

Semen retention might just be the best self-improvement technique you've never heard about. However, this practice has been around a very long time. It has its origins in the ancient practices of traditional Chinese Medicine and Indian Ayurvedic healing. Before we delve into the history of semen retention, let's first understand more about what we're talking about.

WHAT IS SEMEN RETENTION?
Semen retention is quite simply the act of avoiding ejaculation. You can do this by avoiding masturbation and sex altogether for specified periods of time. If you want to continue being sexually active, the other option is to separate your orgasm from ejaculation. In this way, you can experience the pleasure and connction of sex, including orgasm, without experiencing an ejaculation. This is called a "dry orgasm."

The first thing that likely crosses your mind when hearing about this is why? Why do this? You might be surprised to hear that there are actually numerous benefits to this ancient practice. We'll go into more depth on the benefits of semen retention in subsequent chapters, but here is a brief list of how it can help you become a better version of yourself:

- Increases productivity
- Increases motivation
- Boosts your income potential
- Increases focus
- Boosts self-confidence
- Increases your energy
- Boosts your libido
- Strengthens your immune system
- Sharpens your memory
- Makes you more of a risk-taker
- Helps you sleep
- Relieves depression
- Deepens your voice
- Gives you stronger hair
- Improves your self-control

There are even scientific studies that have documented the following benefits of semen retention:

- An increase in testosterone levels.
- An increase in the brain's androgen receptors (ARs) that facilitate the flow of male hormones through your body.
- Decrease in dopamine levels — that's a feel-good neurochemical that plays a key role in addictive behaviors.
- Decrease in prolactin levels — that's a hormone which prompts the production of sperm, but too much of it can interfere with the proper function of the testicles.

- Increase in serotonin levels — that's a neurochemical which helps to prevent depression and boosts mental health.

The idea behind semen retention is that you can reorient the energy involved in sexual pleasure, culminating in ejaculation, to boost performance in other areas of life. Many who practice semen retention believe it increases both physical and spiritual energy. In short, sexual energy can be harnessed and redirected as a powerful creative force in other areas of your life.

You can use it as a driver for your creative, professional and personal success. What's more, you can do this without sacrificing the pleasure of the sexual experience, if you so choose to. Let's take a closer look at where this practice originated and who has used it successfully to improve their life.

HISTORIC ORIGINS OF SEMEN RETENTION

In traditional Chinese Medicine, ancient texts speak about three vital forces of life. These are Jing, or essence, Qi, or air, and Shen, or spirit.

Jing is conceived of as the life force that nourishes, fuels and cools the body. It is believed that everyone is born with a fixed amount of Jing, although it is possible to attain more from certain foods and various forms of stimulation such as exercise and meditation.

Jing is considered important for longevity, and the most concentrated form of Jing is in semen. By releasing semen out of the body, therefore, you are losing some of your Jing. It's kind of like mojo, and you don't want to lose your mojo!

The loss of Jing, according to the ancient texts, results in disease, premature aging, fatigue and deterioration in general.

While ejaculation results in the loss of Jing, the union of two people in sexual communication allows a man to transform some of his Jing into Qi, thereby replenishing his life force. Thus, sex is considered a healthy act that replenishes the life force, but ejaculation itself represents a loss of life energy.

According to this belief, by practicing semen retention techniques, men can benefit energetically and spiritually from the union with another while simultaneously retaining their life force. In other words, you don't have to sacrifice your life force to experience sexual pleasure.

In the ancient Hindu texts, there are similar ideas to that of traditional Chinese Medicine. Ayurvedic texts describe semen as derived from blood. In fact, one drop of semen is said to be elaborated from 80 drops of blood (modern western medicine notes that it takes 40 drops of blood to manufacture one drop of semen).

Semen is said to be pervasive throughout the body, much in the same way that sugar is for sugar cane and fat is for butter. When you remove fat from butter, the butter is thin and weak, and the same is true for semen in the body. Weakness results from wastage. In the 12th century Sanskrit text, the Yogaśāstra, the loss of semen was described as follows:

"Falling of semen brings death; preservation of semen gives life. Semen is the real vitality in man. It is the hidden treasure for man. It imparts Brahma Tejas (*the rays of the Lord*) to the face and strength to the intellect."

In Hindu mysticism, the root chakra, located at the base of the spine, is believed to be where the Kundalini Shakti — or your true power — resides. This is associated with creative sexual energy, and ultimately responsible for all of creation. Additionally, it is considered to be the agent of all change.

When the Kundalini energy rises throughout your body, it brings about physical and mental strength and potency. Semen is a primary component of this power. In this practice, as in many Taoist sects, semen retention is a spiritual practice, often referred to as "galvanizing energy".

Losing ejaculatory fluids is akin to losing vital life force, and thus, semen retention enhances the spiritual experience of galvanizing your energies because it keeps the life force inside you. In fact, some Taoists argue that you should never ejaculate, while others have developed a specific formula for the maximum amount of regular ejaculations you can have and still stay healthy. Either way, they emphatically believe that you have to preserve semen to conserve the life essence — the Jing.

WHO DOES THIS?

You might be surprised to find out that many famous and highly successful people have practiced semen retention.

Napoleon Hill wrote about the practice in his book, *Think and Grow Rich*. He noted that sexual desire is a major driver of successful characteristics like imagination, willpower, persistence, courage and creativity. Even men who are unsuccessful in other parts of their lives can marshall these traits when harnessing their sexual desire.

Thus, if the energy that promotes these characteristics can be harnessed and redirected to other aspects of life, it can be a powerful creative force for any form of professional and personal development, says Hill.

Given the list of successful men who have used the technique, it's hard to argue he's wrong.

Here is a list of some famous athletes who have practiced

semen retention:

- Muhammad Ali — boxer
- Mike Tyson — boxer
- Saido Takamori — considered the most influential Samurai in Japanese history
- David Haye — world heavyweight boxing champion
- Manny Pacquiao — eight-division world champion boxer
- Martin "Farmer" Burns — world champion wrestler
- Rickson Gracie — mixed martial arts and Jiu-Jitsu legend
- The Great Gama — undefeated world champion wrestler, champion of world wrestling between 1910 and 1928

Sports not your thing? Here's a few famous scientists and business people who have practiced semen retention:

- Sigmund Freud
- Sir Isaac Newton
- Steve Jobs
- Nikola Tesla

Here's a few philosophers you might have heard about, too:

- Plato
- Socrates
- The Dalai Lama
- Pythagoras
- Swami Vivekananda

Now, here are a few creative innovators you might know who have used semen retention:

- Michelangelo
- Leo Tolstoy
- Miles Davis
- Kanye West
- 50 Cent
- Mark Wahlberg

HOW IS IT DONE?
We'll go into some specific techniques in later chapters, but as an introduction, semen retention is typically achieved in two ways.

The first is abstinence, and while that can mean abstaining from masturbation and sex altogether, it can also mean abstaining for periods in between your sexual activity.

The other method involves muscle control while having sex. Basically, you have to learn how to have an orgasm without ejaculating. Sounds tricky, doesn't it? But it's really not that difficult. It just takes a little practice. You want to begin by doing some Kegel exercises. Your Kegel muscles are pelvic floor muscles, and by flexing them right before ejaculation, you can have what's called a "dry orgasm."

To strengthen your Kegel muscles, you can start by tightening the muscles that prevent you from passing gas or urinating midstream. You use the same muscles for the actions necessary to prevent ejaculation.

To strengthen the Kegel muscles, you simply contract those muscles and hold for three seconds and then relax them for three seconds. Do this several times a day. You'll also want to practice contracting only those muscles while keeping your buttocks, thighs and abdomen relaxed and while breathing freely.

Once strengthened, you'll use the same technique as an orgasm is near to prevent ejaculation. You can also practice this by masturbating. At first, your timing might be off, but keep at it, and you'll get it down. We'll go through all this in more detail later in the book.

WHAT ARE THE SPIRITUAL BENEFITS?
Aside from the physical benefits of semen retention, many people believe it has significant spiritual benefits.

As we've discussed, the ancient Far Eastern texts believe that sperm is a major component of your vital life force. With the retention of semen, those philosophies hold that you can experience a greater sense of life purpose and overall harmony. They also argue that you develop stronger and deeper emotional bonds in your relationships. This brings about a greater sense of life satisfaction.

Kundalini energy is believed to reside at the base of the spine, where the root chakra is said to be located. It is considered a feminine energy, but when awakened, it rises up through the body to the head where the energy of Lord Shiva is located. At this point, the masculine and feminine unite, which leads to a loss of the sense of duality. In other words, you wake to your own divinity. It is considered the purest ecstasy of union. The root chakra is also associated with sexual energy, and the retention of semen allows for that energy to be redirected into a Kundalini awakening — which can power your life in any direction where you focus the energy.

WHAT ABOUT RELATIONSHIP BENEFITS?
Semen retention actually has numerous benefits for your relationship. First, if your partner understands your reasons

for doing it and is supportive, you can both reap the benefits of this practice. It can create a stronger bond between the two of you as the focus is no longer on an end goal. It can also increase the anticipation of the sexual experience, and it can increase the intensity of the orgasms that you do have.

Also, because you're focusing on controlling your sexual experience, you can then concentrate on pleasing your partner. That will increase your sexual stamina, and a big bonus is that you can also have the potential to experience multiple orgasms (without ejaculation). It's not just for the ladies anymore.

You'll also experience more self-control and a greater sense of body awareness. This will definitely improve your sexual technique. Finally, semen retention also improves the quality of your sperm. They will have higher motility, and you'll have more of them. That's good news if you are trying to conceive.

In summary, you can begin to see numerous benefits from semen retention.

You'll experience a greater sense of self-control, more intense sexual pleasure with greater stamina, improved fertility, a strong sense of self-awareness, a boost in energy, a better immune system, and a stronger sense of spiritual connection to the world around you.

You'll also have more motivation and energy for achieving your life goals as well as creating stronger relationship bonds. That all adds up to greater personal and professional life satisfaction. So, are you ready to give it a try? If so, let's dive right in!

CHAPTER SUMMARY
In this chapter, we've discussed the basics of semen retention.

Specifically, we've covered the following subjects:

- What is semen retention
- What are some physical benefits
- The mystical origins of the practice
- Famous and successful people who practice semen retention
- The spiritual and relationship benefits of semen retention

In the next chapter, you will learn everything you always wanted to know about semen.

2

EVERYTHING YOU NEED TO KNOW ABOUT SEMEN

Before we dive deeper into the history and ancient wisdom regarding semen retention, it's important first to understand semen's biology. To that end, let's explore the nutrients and energy it contains and how it is replenished. Here, you'll learn everything you always wanted to know about semen but were afraid to ask!

Just so you know, this chapter is necessarily quite dense and we go into the biological details. You can skip ahead and get to the more practical aspects of the book if you wish. But if you stay you will be armed with detailed medical information as to why semen is so precious. In fact, you'll know just as much as most doctors about the topic!

Let's first look at how your body creates it.

SEMEN PRODUCTION
You might have never thought about this before, but semen isn't just simply produced in the testicles. In fact, the process

involves your brain, your endocrine system and the autonomic nervous system, as well as your testicles. In a sense, it takes a village to produce semen, and the village in this scenario is your entire body.

The process starts in your brain, in an area called the hypothalamus. The hypothalamus is attached to a gland called the pituitary gland. This pea-sized gland is known as the master gland because it directly produces, or initiates the production of, every hormone in your body.

Hormones are like the body's messengers. They are essentially the way that different parts of your body communicate with one another. There are a number of hormones involved in semen production. The three hormones we'll talk about are the Gonadotropin-Releasing Hormone (GnRH), the Luteinizing Hormone (LH) and the Follicle Stimulating Hormone (FSH).

The semen production process begins when the hypothalamus secretes GnRH, causing the pituitary gland to release both LH and FSH. The body begins to produce GnRH during puberty.

Once LH and FSH are released, they go to the testes where they effectively send a message to specialized cells located there: Leydig and Sertoli cells. When the Leydig cells receive the LH message from the pituitary gland, they begin to convert cholesterol into testosterone.

You've probably heard of testosterone, but you may not know what it is exactly and what it does. Basically, it's another hormone — that is, another messenger — that enters the Sertoli cells. Once testosterone enters these Sertoli cells, it triggers cell division known as mitosis and meiosis.

You might remember something about mitosis and meiosis from high school biology. These are the processes of cell division. With mitosis, you basically get a clone of the "parent" cell, and this is the division process that every cell in your body goes through, except for the sex cells — that is, the sperm and the egg.

The cell division that produces sperm and an egg is known as meiosis. With meiosis, instead of a clone of the parent cell, the "daughter" cells produced by this process only have one-half of the genetic material that the parent cell had. Why? Because that cell with one-half of the genetic material will meet up with another cell where it will get the other half of the genetic material needed to produce a new life.

When sperm is created, stem cells in the Sertoli cells first divide by mitosis. They then begin the process of meiosis, and the resulting spermatozoa (the technical name for sperm) begins to mature. As with any baby, infant sperm have to have the proper environment to mature. The incubation chambers for these baby sperm are called seminiferous tubules. The walls of these tubules are lined with mucus, and this is where the Sertoli cells attach. The Sertoli cells actually form a tight tissue barrier that keeps harmful products, like bacteria, from entering the incubation chamber, and it keeps fluids inside the chamber from leaking out. This tight barrier is called the Blood-Testis Barrier (BTB).

It's important to keep a concentrated level of testosterone in the fluid within the incubation chamber for the sperm to mature. The problem is that much of the liquid in the chamber is water, and testosterone is liposoluble, meaning it concentrates in fat rather than water. That means it would be difficult to achieve the levels of concentration necessary for testosterone to keep the developing sperm healthy were it not for the other hormone we mentioned, FSH. FSH enters the Sertoli cells and causes them to release a protein called the Androgen Binding Protein (ABP). That binds the testosterone molecules so that it can remain highly concentrated in the watery liquid of the tubules.

All of this activity in your seminiferous tubules requires a specific temperature to occur. That's why the testicles are located externally. If they were up inside the body, the temperature would be too high, so they must hang outside the body in the wrinkled scrotal sac. It's wrinkled because it needs to adapt — stretch out and relax again — as the muscles within the testes contract and relax in an effort to regulate the temperature.

If it's a warm day, the testicles hang lower, and if it's cold outside, they are pulled up closer to the body so that their temperature will always remain at around 93.2 degrees Fahrenheit (34 degrees Celsius), the ideal temperature for sperm production to occur. This is lower than the normal body temperature of 98.6 degrees Fahrenheit (37 degrees Celsius), which is why they can't be inside the body.

The product of this activity is a fully formed "spermatozoon" with a head, a body and a tail. We're still not done, though, because we don't yet have semen. There's more to semen than just sperm cells. To understand how we get semen, we must understand the erection and ejaculation process.

ERECTION & EJACULATION

The system that controls erection and ejaculation is called the autonomic nervous system. If you read that as automatic instead of autonomic, it's okay — you're not far off. In fact, the autonomic nervous system controls your body's unconscious processes, like breathing. You don't have to think about breathing; you just do it. It's automatic, and if you try to hold your breath until you die, you can't do it. You'll pass out. The autonomic nervous system will take over, and you'll start breathing again. This same system controls both erection and ejaculation.

The autonomic nervous system is made up of two different parts: the sympathetic nervous system and the parasympathetic nervous system. These two parts are like two sides of the same coin. Your sympathetic nervous system is your "fight or flight" nervous system. When stimulated, it gets your body ready for action so that you can survive an attack. That means your heart rate increases, as does your breathing rate. There are a number of other physical responses to the hormones released when this system is activated.

The parasympathetic nervous system is the other side of the coin. It calms you down after the excitement has passed. You can think of it as your "chill and relax" system. These systems work in co-ordination to produce an erection and ejaculation.

When a man is aroused, the parasympathetic nervous system is stimulated to relax certain muscles. The relaxation of these muscles allows blood to engorge the tissues of the penis, resulting in an erection. The parasympathetic nervous system also sends an excitatory message to the vas deferens, the seminal vesicles and the prostate gland. The vas deferens is the tube through which the semen travels to exit the body, and the seminal vesicles and prostate gland are the structures that produce seminal fluid.

When a man has an orgasm, the sympathetic nervous system takes over. It ultimately causes a constriction of the blood vessels that engorge the penile tissues with blood. That cuts off the blood flow into those tissues, resulting in a loss of the erection. But as the orgasm is happening, the sympathetic nervous system also causes a structure called the epididymis to contract and squeeze out those mature sperm cells in the seminiferous tubules. This pushes the sperm into the vas deferens. The vas deferens also contracts to push the sperm outside via the urethra, which is the tube through which urine passes. Right before the sperm enters the urethra, a ring of muscle (sphincter) contracts to close off the part of the urethra coming from the bladder. That way, sperm can't travel up into the bladder. When semen is ejaculated, it travels at an approximate velocity of 11 miles per hour.

It would be a difficult ride indeed, were it not for the seminal fluid. It is the combination of the sperm and the seminal fluid that is called semen. The seminal fluid is also what nourishes the sperm and protects them from the acidic environment of the vagina so that they can enter the uterus to seek out an egg. It is because of the seminal fluid that sperm can live for approximately 72 hours after ejaculation. But what is this fluid, and where is it produced?

SEMINAL FLUID
That structure that squeezes the sperm into the vas deferens — the epididymis — also secretes sodium, glyceryl phosphorylcholine and potassium. These join the sperm as they enter the vas deferens. The sperm pass through the vas deferens and enter a storage area called the ampulla. The ampulla adds fructose — a type of sugar — to the sperm and a yellowish fluid called ergothioneine, which decreases or removes oxygen from the chemical compounds present.

Finally, the seminal vesicles and prostate gland add what's called a pre-ejaculatory fluid to the mix. All of these components of the seminal fluid make up approximately 60 percent of the total semen volume, and their job is to nourish the sperm and protect them. Let's take a closer look at the seminal vesicles and prostate gland structures involved in seminal fluid production.

THE PROSTATE & COWPER'S GLANDS
Cowper's gland, named after William Cowper, the 17th-century surgeon who discovered it, is a pea-sized gland located beneath the prostate gland in the area where the internal parts of the penis begin. As a man ejaculates, this gland adds clear, thick fluids that act as a lubricant and help to flush the urethra before the ejaculation of the semen. These fluids make the semen less watery and account for approximately 5 percent of the total seminal fluid.

The prostate gland is probably the best-known gland in the male reproductive tract because of prostate cancer. It is a gland about the size of a walnut, and it is located between the penis and the bladder. It also adds fluid secretions to the sperm as it is being ejaculated.

The gland itself actually surrounds the urethra, so if it becomes overgrown, it can decrease the diameter of the urethra and slow the flow of urine. That's why older men sometimes take a long time to urinate. The fluid from the prostate, called pre-ejaculate, can be clear or milky-white, and is slightly acidic.

The fluid contains citric acid and certain enzymes. Enzymes cause an action to occur, and in this case, the action is to split proteins. The fluid produced by the prostate also contains sodium, zinc, calcium and potassium. Approximately 15 to 30 percent of the seminal fluid is this substance produced by the prostate gland.

SEMINAL VESICLES

The seminal vesicles are actually two small glands located inside the pelvis. The fluid they produce and secrete into the ejaculatory tract includes fructose, citric acid, potassium, proteins, phosphorus and prostaglandins. The fructose provides a source of energy for the sperm when it is outside the man's body, and the prostaglandins are lipids or fatty substances that support fertilization. Basically, these make the cervix's mucus lining a bit more "welcoming" for the sperm. They also help to move the sperm towards the egg. The seminal vesicles produce approximately 65 to 75 percent of the seminal fluid.

At this point, I'm sure you're starting to get the idea that this process is a lot more complicated than how we're used to thinking about it. It truly takes a village, and that village has to be well-nourished for the entire process to run smoothly and produce healthy, fertile sperm. That's why it's important to understand the essential vitamins and minerals required for healthy spermatogenesis (sperm production).

ESSENTIAL VITAMINS & MINERALS FOR SPERM PRODUCTION

There are a number of nutrients that are essential to the process of sperm production. Let's look at the role of each of these.

- **Zinc**: This is one of the main components found in the testes, sperm and in the semen. It is thirty times more concentrated in the semen than it is in the blood. It is not produced by the body, and therefore must be included as part of a healthy diet. It is found in meat, dairy products, eggs, and legumes like quinoa, chickpeas and lentils.

Zinc is crucial for the proper replication of genetic material required for healthy mitosis and meiosis. It is necessary to maintain good levels of proteins, like the Androgen Binding Protein that keeps testosterone concentration at proper levels. That's vital for the maturation process of the sperm in the incubating chambers. Some research (Cheah and Yang, 2011) has shown that a deficiency in zinc is associated with a lower sperm count as well as a decrease in testicular weight and shrinking of the seminiferous tubules.

Zinc is also found in the sperm's tail. It helps distribute energy so the sperm cell can swim and navigate through obstacles. In the seminal fluid, it is also an antioxidant that cleans up the sperms' waste products as they utilize fructose to make energy. Were it not for the zinc, those waste products could harm the sperm cells.

- *Selenium*: Selenium is another vital mineral for sperm production. It is found in shiitake mushrooms, oatmeal, tofu, shellfish and lean pork. Its main function is to act as an antioxidant. It is present in large concentrations in the incubation chambers of the testes. There, it protects stem cells as they engage in cell division (mitosis and meiosis). These processes require a lot of energy, and the utilization of that energy produces a lot of waste products, known as free radicals.

The stem cells are extremely vulnerable to these waste products, and that's why they need to be protected. Once the stem cells mature into sperm cells, they no longer require this protection, but they're not done with the selenium. It actually becomes the midpiece or body of the sperm cell. That's why a selenium deficiency will decrease the sperm count. Without it, the stem cells don't survive during cell division. Moreover, a deficiency of selenium can affect the sperm's motility, that is, its ability to move. The sperm's midpiece is its engine, and without an engine, they can't move.

- ***Vitamins***: There are also some important vitamins required for sperm production. These include B12, A, E and C. Vitamin B12 is found in animal products and fermented vegetables. Carrots, broccoli, cantaloupe and squash all contain Vitamin A. Vitamin E is found in spinach, almonds, sunflower seeds and broccoli. Lastly, Vitamin C is found in citrus fruits, tomatoes, peppers, cauliflower, cabbage, and yes, you guessed it, broccoli.

The functions of these vitamins vary. B12 is necessary for cell replication and division by helping produce DNA and RNA, the body's genetic blueprints. A deficiency in this vitamin affects the division of the sperm cells, which reduces the overall sperm count (Cheah and Yang, 2011). Vitamins C and E act as antioxidants to protect the internal testicular tissues and the cells' DNA from oxidative stress as waste products are produced. A deficiency in either of these vitamins causes mutations in the testicular tissues and either decreased sperm counts or dysfunctional sperm. Finally, Vitamin A activates certain genes that are necessary for normal cell function.

- ***Macronutrients***: Carbohydrates, lipids and proteins are macronutrients that also play a role in sperm production. Lipids, or fats, carry liposoluble vitamins and act as a source of fuel for the process. Cell membranes are made of lipids, and the sperm cell membranes affect the way they interact with their environment. They need to be healthy to ingest the necessary nutrients to function properly. Carbohydrates are another fuel source for the sperm cells, and the Androgen Binding Protein (ABP) is a protein that increases testosterone concentration in the seminiferous tubules.

DEPLETION & REPLENISHMENT OF SPERM

The whole process of spermatogenesis takes an average of 64 to 74 days from start to finish. This means that it can take about two months for your sperm cells to mature in the incubating chamber inside your testes.

After the maturation period, sperm cells are pushed out into the epididymis. It takes an additional 14 days for sperm to fully mature in the epididymis. That means it takes nearly three months for the whole cycle to be concluded.

Seminal fluid is a bit different. This substance is more readily available since it is replenished every two days. Although it is produced quicker, it still uses resources to replenish it. Throughout these processes, your body is investing energy in the form of glycogen and fructose. That's in addition to the energy required to make the hormonal messages needed to trigger the processes in the first place.

Thus, sperm takes longer to replenish than seminal fluid, which may be why people are under the impression that sperm can't run out. In reality, it's possible to ejaculate with a high concentration of seminal fluid but a low sperm count or quality. It is possible, therefore, to deplete your sperm. Now that you know that it takes about two to three months for the process of replenishment to take place, you might wonder if there could be other areas of your life that might benefit from these resources.

When thinking about the processes of cell division and new cell growth, it is important to view it from an economic perspective. The body has a certain amount of resources that are distributed to different processes, such as maintaining your current metabolic processes, helping your immune system fight off infections and new cell growth. You can always produce energy itself; however, there are more finite resources involved here, such as the essential nutrients we've discussed, which can be depleted. That's a key way in which semen retention can be beneficial. It can redirect energetic resources to other areas of your body, and the resulting energy can act as jet fuel for your success in different areas of your life.

With this understanding of semen production and the energetic requirements for the process, it's possible to look at ways in which you can utilize those resources in other areas of your life. It's an ancient process, and we'll look at its origins in the next chapter.

By the way, well done if you've made it to the end of this chapter! It wasn't always the easiest reading, but now I'm sure your understanding of what we're dealing with at a biological level has skyrocketed.

CHAPTER SUMMARY

In this chapter, we've discussed the process of semen production (or spermatogenesis). Specifically, we've discussed the following topics:

- How sperm are produced

- The hormones involved in sperm production
- What's involved in erection and ejaculation
- The production of seminal fluid
- The necessary vitamins and minerals for spermatogenesis
- The depletion and replenishment of sperm

In the next chapter, you will learn more in-depth about what the ancient wisdom says about semen retention.

3

ANCIENT WISDOM ON SEMEN RETENTION

This book might be the first time you're hearing about semen retention, but it's not a new concept. It might seem that way because the internet allows for much more rapid communication, particularly on subjects that might have previously been considered taboo. Semen retention, however, is an ancient practice. It has, in fact, been practiced for centuries. Let's look a little more deeply at the origins and wisdom behind this "trend".

CONCEPT OF LIFE ENERGY
The ancient wisdom surrounding the practice of semen retention all speaks of a life energy that exists in your body, and it is often believed to be particularly concentrated in the semen. That's not necessarily surprising, considering the role that semen plays in the creation of life. As the ancient philosophies hold, it is a thriving, expanding energetic force that is evident in nature's design. Traditional Chinese Medicine practitioners

refer to your life force as Qi (pronounced chee), and ancient Hindu texts call it Prana.

Ancient alchemists believed that this life energy is a combination of electric and magnetic forces running through all creation. Moreover, many of these ancient traditions hold that there are centers in your body, called chakras, where the energy concentrates and circulates in a kind of whirlpool pattern before it passes through channels in your body, called meridians, to the various organ systems.

The concepts of Qi or Prana are based on what is called the subtle or spiritual body, but despite the spiritual nature of this energy, it has very real effects on your physical body as well. Both Qi and Prana mean breath, and this is reflective of the way that both Chinese Taoists and Indian Tantra practitioners believe that we "ingest" this energy, that is, through breathing. This is actually congruent with western medicine, given that your body needs oxygen to make energy, and you receive oxygen through breathing. Thus, as with many things, the ancient philosophies are one step ahead of science.

Qi and Prana, however, have deeper, more spiritual connotations as well. As the so-called Kundalini energy awakens at the base of your spine in the root chakra and rises through the other chakras, it finally arrives at the crown chakra. The crown chakra sits just above the crown of your head, and when the Kundalini energy reaches that point, you experience an awakening into the oneness of the universe. You merge with the divine, so to speak. We can call it enlightenment.

The energy of Qi or Prana is more than simply spiritual, though. It is also creative, and these philosophies further hold that the element that creates the spark of life exists in the air around us, but it can be harnessed and stored in your sperm.

From there, it can be used to create new life. It is also possible to utilize that creative energy in other areas of your life.

TRANSMUTATION & ALCHEMY

The practice of semen retention is based on the principle of transmutation. This idea originated in alchemical schools of thought that date back to the Hellenistic Period. This is the time period between the death of Alexander the Great in 323 BC and the rise of the Roman Empire around 31 BC.

During the Hellenestic Period, many Greek philosophers became interested in the Egyptian schools of mystery. It was as a result of this interest that the combination of Greek and Egyptian philosophies, which came to be known as alchemy, was born. In fact, there is a philosophy known as Hermeticism that was developed out of this union and is responsible for documenting the principles of alchemy.

Hermes Trismegistus was a symbolic figure combining the Greek god Hermes with the Egyptian god Thoth. These deities were believed to bear messages in each of their religions. Hermes Trismegistus was the author's name on the *Emerald Tablet*, the first scripture that discussed transmutation. In reality, the writings in the *Emerald Tablet* are likely older traditions that had been passed down orally before that time, and it is from these traditions that the alchemical principles were derived. The *Emerald Tablet* specifically lists seven alchemical principles, but two are important for our purposes here.

One alchemical principle that is relevant for semen retention is the principle of vibration. It is the third alchemical principle in the *Emerald Tablet*. It basically states that everything has a vibrational frequency, and because the vibrational frequencies are subject to change, everything is constantly changing. This principle is in line with what western science has discovered as well. It all boils down to energy, and all energy has a frequency. This is a key concept of quantum physics.

The other alchemical principle important for our discussion of semen retention is the fifth principle of rhythm. This states that the universe has a rhythm. It is cyclical, and that if you can attune your own energy to the rhythmic patterns of the universe, you can use those rhythms to your advantage. Of course, science has also established that cycles govern the processes of life. So, what does this have to do with semen retention?

The concept of transmutation basically involves the transformation of one thing into another. The story goes that ancient alchemists were obsessed with turning lead into gold, but many people interpret this as a metaphor. In fact, Pythagoras, a Greek philosopher, taught his followers about what would later be realized as semen's alchemical properties. He knew that semen was a vital fluid that was substantively similar to the tissues of the brain, and he understood the role it played in creative energy. He taught his followers that such energy is best conserved for the brain rather than expended in a wasteful manner. That doesn't necessarily mean being celibate, just not being wasteful.

A Pythagorean physician named Alemeon also claimed that semen, if properly conserved, would be transformed into nourishment for the brain. They were not the only philosophers of their time to think like that. In fact, Aristotle, Plato, Leonardo da Vinci, Isaac Newton and Beethoven are all examples of philosophers, creatives and highly successful people who practiced the concepts of semen retention. This is how transmutation applies to semen. You can harness this vital, creative life force and direct its energy toward other applications in your life. This doesn't mean it can't also be used for its purpose to create life and allow for sexual pleasure, but if it is not wasted, you can use that powerful energetic force in other areas as well.

To understand how this principle works, let's take the example of anger. Anger is a fiery emotion that is born in the amygdala of your brain. That's the part of your brain that gets activated by fear. The sympathetic nervous system — remember that's the fight or flight nervous system — stimulates this area of the brain, which causes the release of cortisol and adrenaline, among other hormones. The purpose of these hormones is to focus your attention and prepare your body for action. This alert state often takes the form of anger, which can be very helpful if you need to increase aggression, fight for your life or fend off a predator.

Alchemists teach that this fiery emotion of anger can be transformed or transmuted into passion. It might be a passion for justice — anger fuelled the anti-apartheid and women's liberation movement. It can also be a creative passion. In this way, what can sometimes be a destructive energy force can be transformed into creative energy for making the world a better place. You might be wondering exactly how semen can be transformed, so let's look at the components of semen and how they are similar to those found in the brain, which is the root of all of our actions.

SEMEN AND THE BRAIN

The brain and semen both contain high levels of chemicals such as sodium, magnesium, and lecithin, but one of the most important chemicals for our purposes here is phosphorus. The name phosphorus means "light-bringer," and in fact, phosphorus does produce a fiery reaction when administered internally. It stimulates the nervous system in a powerful way. Moreover, it's essential for life since it's an important component of DNA and other genetic material. Its action did not go unnoticed by early alchemists, either. In fact, phosphorus is the "philosopher's stone" that is the central symbol of alchemy. It is meant to symbolize the light within DNA and in nature.

So, the concept is rather simple. Because semen is high in phosphorus, if you conserve your semen, you're conserving your phosphorus, and the brain can use it for generating fiery, creative energy. If you waste it, you will lose the opportunity to direct that fiery energy towards your external goals. Conserving it means the brain gets to use it. That doesn't mean you have to refrain from having sex altogether, but the act of sex should be an opportunity to unite two souls; it should be cherished and respected. If you conserve your semen for those sacred unions, at other times, that energy is available for productive uses.

Alchemists weren't the only ones who understood these concepts. There are many similarities between the principles of alchemy and the ideas proposed by Taoists and Tantra yogis. They, too, understood the energetic principles used by alchemists, and they realized how important the proper flow of energy throughout the body is for health and well-being.

They documented their ideas related to energy flow and health in ancient texts like the *Tao Te Ching*, the *Huang Di Nei Jing* and the Hindu Tantras. In these texts, they discussed the flow of energy through the body and the effect of blocked energy on the various organs. They recognized the association between this energetic flow and physical, mental, emotional and spiritual health. Furthermore, they recognized how stimulating this energy could attune your vibrational frequencies and energetic rhythm to what you hope to attract into your life. Let's take a look at what they said specifically about semen.

TAOISM & QI

Tao (pronounced "Dao") can be translated into the "path" or the "way". Taoism teaches that every stone, every leaf and every part of the universe or nature is God. Everything is part of a larger energetic system, and thus, that energy can be directed in myriad ways. You can live in a conscious manner by showing gratitude for everything around you. Grounding yourself in the present moment, they say, relieves all suffering.

With regard to sex, Taoism teaches that love is a manifestation of our sex drive. To put it another way, it is our sex drive transmuted. Our sex drive is much like lead, and love is gold in the alchemical metaphor. By love, we don't only mean romantic love, though that's included as well, but love as passion, the passion you have for life. It's a motivating force that drives you to care about yourself and the world around you.

Taoism teaches us that we can redirect the creative energy of our sex drive towards other areas in life as well. You can use this drive to be passionate about work, passionate about enjoying the experiences life has to offer, passionate about justice, and passionate about taking care of your health. Taoism and alchemists propose that we need only synchronize ourselves with life's rhythms and use the natural flow of energy to our advantage.

The question then becomes how to synchronize yourself

with the natural flow of the universe. Tao philosophy proposes that you do this by aligning yourself with nature's creative and expansive tendencies, but what does that actually mean for you?

Self-actualization — reaching your true potential — and discovering your purpose in life are the human version of creativity and expansion. This is how you align yourself with the flow of the universe. If you don't strive to live your purpose, you'll likely feel unfulfilled in life, and that can lead to any number of maladies, including depression, obesity, anxiety and addiction. But how do you tap into your creative potential? This is where semen retention comes into play.

As we mentioned before, our sex drive is a powerful force that motivates many decisions we make in life. You would be surprised by how much of what people do in life is motivated by sex. This is due to nature's creative tendency. It wants us to procreate and continue to thrive. This is the driving force behind evolution. In fact, the entire principle of natural selection is about procreation. It's not about how long you live, although you must live long enough to reproduce, and it's not even about being healthy, although there too, you must be healthy enough to reproduce. It's all about reproduction. That's the motivating factor behind everything in nature. You must accumulate enough resources to grow, be healthy and reach reproductive age. From there, you must have the resources to attract a mate and support offspring. Thus, your instincts, and those of all of nature, are geared towards this purpose.

Humans have added a layer of culture on top of this drive. For example, money is something we give cultural value to, but it really translates into resources. You can buy shelter, food and anything else you need to attract a mate and reproduce.

But what if you took this instinctual drive and used it more consciously to achieve your goals? What if you were able to take that energy and apply it to cultivating your talents and realizing your true potential and purpose in life, and creating meaningful relationships? That is the "way" described in Taoism.

It's similar to what is expressed in the Hindu Tantras as well. The main difference is that the tantric texts are more spiritual in nature. They emphasize using your life force to achieve enlightenment, whereas Taoism focuses on the body and your health. Still, both are based on the concept of universal oneness through consciousness.

Thus, when we realign ourselves to the vibrational frequency and rhythms of the universe, we can easily redirect energetic forces to create anything we wish to generate in our lives. It is a matter of transmuting the energetic forces into the changes we wish to see in our lived reality. In Hinduism, the union of male and female energetic forces creates enlightenment. In a way, the energy is transmuted into enlightenment.

In Ayurvedic texts, semen is likened to the essence of a tree. The tree draws that essence from the earth and then circulates to every part of the tree, imparting color and life to the leaves and flowers. Semen, called Veerya, similarly gives color and vitality to your body and the different organs within it. This seminal energy is considered to be the secret to good health, and someone who wastes it, it is said, will be unable to achieve either physical, mental, moral or spiritual development. This vital life force — Veerya — when preserved, is described as having the capacity to open the doors to God's realm as well as to the higher achievements you hope to attain in life.

To put it simply, transmutation of the energy in semen is the process of converting sexual energy into some other motivation, energy or drive. When you express your sexual energy by having sex, you dissipate your energy with that act. It leaves the body through the sex organ. But you can redirect it upward into your higher energy centers, that is, those chakras that circulate Qi or Jing.

The sexual energy, when redirected, rises through the chakras where it has effects on your physical and mental health, and capabilities. For example, the solar plexus chakra above the sacral and root chakras is associated with willpower. If a person lacks willpower, it's an indicator that they're losing sexual energy because it is leaking out of their body through excessive sex or masturbation.

They can also lose this energy simply by thoughts associated with desire. It says in the Bible that a man who thinks lustful thoughts has already committed adultery in his heart, and that's in line with what we're referring to here. Even thoughts associated with desire expend your sexual energy. But they're not the only kinds of thoughts that do so. If you worry a lot or tend to overthink things, that, too, expends sexual energy.

If, on the other hand, you can channel your sexual energy by conserving it into other areas of your life, like your career, then you increase your willpower and transmute that energy into achieving your goals in life. When you do this, you align your energetic frequency and rhythms to those found in nature.

We've been discussing what the ancient texts say about semen retention and how it can be beneficial for your health and spirituality. In the next chapter, we'll cover specific benefits of this practice and discuss the scientific evidence for those benefits.

CHAPTER SUMMARY

In this chapter, we've discussed what the ancient texts say about semen and its conservation. Specifically, we've discussed the following topics:

- The concept of life energy
- Transmutation and alchemy
- Taoism, Qi and semen retention
- The Hindu Tantras, Ayurvedic concepts and semen retention

4

WHY SEMEN RETENTION IS SO BENEFICIAL

In this chapter, we'll discuss a number of benefits of semen retention related to your emotional, physical and mental health. Specifically, we'll examine benefits in the following areas:

- Boosts confidence
- Higher energy
- More self-control
- Sharp memory
- Strong hair
- Deep voice
- Relieves depression
- Boosts libido
- Makes you a risk-taker
- Improves sleep
- Boosts your immune system
- Increases your attractiveness
- Awakens your root chakra
- Improves athletic performance

- Makes you happier
- Gives you more time for other things

Let's take a look at each of these benefits individually.

BOOSTS CONFIDENCE

Let's begin with how semen retention can help improve your self-confidence and self-esteem.

You might have heard that most of your sexual pleasure happens in your brain. It's true; your brain is highly involved in the process. Each time you ejaculate, your brain gives you a shot of dopamine. That's the brain's feel-good neurochemical that is associated with feelings of pleasure. In reality, dopamine doesn't make you feel good, per se. It's only a messenger. It's what's called a neurotransmitter that sends messages between nerve cells.

Dopamine is part of the Catecholamine family of chemicals, and it runs along dopamine pathways in parts of the brain associated with reward-motivated behavior. That means that when you perceive the possibility of a particular reward for any kind of behavior, your brain produces dopamine along these pathways. The dopamine itself doesn't give you pleasure. Instead, it motivates you to take actions that will result in a pleasurable outcome.

Dopamine is transmitted from one nerve cell to another by jumping a gap known as a synapse. On the other side of the synapse is a landing pad known as a receptor, but excessive dopamine production can harm the receptor sites. When that happens, the dopamine can't jump that gap, and your dopamine levels drop as a result.

Low levels of dopamine are associated with low levels of

self-confidence as well as diminished levels of motivation and willpower. Reduced dopamine compounds low self-confidence since it's exponentially more difficult to become confident without motivation.

When you conserve your semen and redirect your sexual energy, you're actually boosting your dopamine levels by not firing it in your brain constantly, and your confidence increases as a result.

HIGHER ENERGY

B12 is a crucial vitamin for your semen. It has numerous beneficial effects on the quality of your sperm. It also increases the functionality of your reproductive organs in general.

Specifically, it decreases the toxicity of homocysteine, which is a type of amino acid; it reduces the levels of nitric oxide; it decreases the oxidative damage done to sperm; and it also decreases the impairment of sperm caused by inflammation. It's contained within your sperm and it is crucial for their stamina. It also helps your body to transform the food you eat into energy that your cells can use. Moreover, it helps keep blood and nerve cells strong and prevents a type of anemia that can cause fatigue. When you ejaculate, you lose vitamin B12, and that can make you feel exhausted.

Abstaining from ejaculation means you don't lose the B12 found in sperm, and you also boost your testosterone levels. In fact, semen retention boosts your testosterone levels by a whopping 45 percent, although it will drop back to normal levels after a few days. High testosterone, like B12, is linked to higher energy levels. Low testosterone causes fatigue, erectile dysfunction and a loss of interest in even having sex.

MORE SELF-CONTROL

Because masturbation stimulates the pleasure and reward centers in the brain, it can create a sensation similar to addiction. That obsessive craving can undermine your willpower and self-control. By refraining from ejaculation, you can make yourself stronger, and you can enhance your self-control. When you have an improved sense of self-control, you also feel more confident in your ability to tackle whatever life throws your way. It's a virtuous circle.

SHARP MEMORY

When you're focused on your sexual desires, whether in the form of self-pleasuring or sex with a partner, it can impair your mental clarity and memory. Remember that phosphorus and zinc are major components of semen, which also keep your brain healthy and sharp. Withholding your semen can increase the power of your memory by retaining these essential nutrients.

STRONG HAIR

Semen contains a protein called keratin. It's the same protein found in your fingernails and hair, and it's essential for their health. It keeps your hair smoother and easier to manage. A decrease in the keratin in your body is associated with hair loss, roughness, dryness and thin hair. Excessive masturbating causes you to lose that valuable keratin, and without keratin, your hair becomes thin and brittle. Additionally, too much self-pleasuring can dry out your scalp and make your head feel itchy because of the lack of keratin. When you practice semen retention, you find that your hair becomes thicker, more lush and your scalp feels better.

DEEP VOICE

As we've mentioned earlier, semen retention boosts your testosterone levels by as much as 45 percent within just one week. That makes your voice deeper, something considered to be an attractive masculine trait.

RELIEVES DEPRESSION

Because semen retention boosts your testosterone levels, it can help to alleviate depression. You need to have optimal levels of testosterone for mental well-being. In fact, people with low levels of testosterone often don't respond to antidepressant medications. When study participants were given testosterone in addition to their medication, they responded well to the combination.

Aside from the physical boost provided by testosterone, there are often problems with people feeling guilty following masturbation. When that happens repeatedly, it trains the brain to respond with frustration and self-reproach each time you masturbate. It's a feedback loop that can have serious negative consequences as it affects your emotions and self-image.

BOOSTS LIBIDO

Your libido is your overall sex drive, which means your desire for sexual activity. People who regularly refrain from masturbation report that their sexual desire increases. They also report that the quality of that desire improves, is deeper and more passionate. This is likely related to increased levels of testosterone. People also report that the increase in self-control they have due to their restraint helps them channel this increased sexual energy into other activities requiring high levels of energy.

MAKES YOU A RISK-TAKER

While there are certainly people who engage in risky behavior and, as a result, pay a high price, what we are talking about here refers more to taking calculated risks that come with big rewards. For example, Steve Jobs, who famously practiced semen retention, took a big risk when he dropped out of college to co-found Apple. His risk paid off, and that's true for many opportunities that come your way in life. They involve significant risk, but they also come with a big payoff. Increased testosterone levels result in taking more bold actions, particularly when it comes to taking financial and professional risks. Many successful entrepreneurs practice semen retention and cite it as a factor in their success.

IMPROVES SLEEP

Low testosterone levels are associated with a reduction in sleep duration, poorer sleep quality, frequently waking up through the night and disturbance while sleeping. Maintaining optimal testosterone levels will improve your overall quality of sleep, and with more and better sleep, you also produce more testosterone. Another virtuous circle in action.

In fact, men who sleep less than five or six hours a night have as much as 10 percent less testosterone in their bodies. That's a big difference that semen retention can help to resolve.

BOOSTS YOUR IMMUNE SYSTEM

Because your semen contains numerous essential vitamins and minerals such as Vitamin C, calcium, magnesium, citric acid, phosphorus, sodium, potassium, zinc, lactic acid and Vitamin B12, among others, it offers tremendous support for your immune system. These nutrients are powerful antioxidants.

Antioxidants work to protect your cells from the damaging effects of free radicals. Free radicals produce inflammation in your body, and inflammation is linked to a number of diseases such as arthritis, cancer, heart disease and diabetes. These essential vitamins and minerals support your immune system's efforts to keep you healthy by helping to reduce inflammation. When you ejecaculate, these nutrients are expelled and your body needs time and resources to build them up again.

INCREASES YOUR ATTRACTIVENESS
This is a big benefit for many men, and if you plan on continuing to have sex even as you practice semen retention, this will be important for you. Because semen retention boosts your testosterone levels and increases your confidence, people find you more attractive. Moreover, the quality of your sexual experiences improves with semen retention, and that makes the connection with your partner deeper and more satisfying. They feel it too, and that makes you even more attractive to them,

Also, semen retention allows you to channel energy into other areas of your life, which increases your success professionally and personally, enhancing your confidence. Sex is a primary motivator for most men, and thus, if you're more attractive, that's a big benefit. Additionally, the more confident you are, the more attractive you are, and that makes you even more confident. It's another positive feedback loop.

AWAKENS YOUR ROOT CHAKRA
Your root chakra is the first chakra. It's located at the base of your spine, and its energy is linked to the earth element. It's also where your Kundalini energy lies and awaits awakening.

Because the root chakra is associated with the earth element, it's also linked to your feelings of being grounded and safe. It's your foundational energy that sets the stage for expansion in your life since it's associated with your physical body and providing nutrients to your tissues. It's also responsible for motivating foundational behaviors like eating, sleeping and procreating. Thus, it is an important factor in both generating and conserving sexual energy.

When conserved, you can direct that energy toward spiritual awakening and expansion, professional success and personal growth. By opening this chakra and keeping it balanced, you help maintain the health of your other chakras as well. Additionally, you can awaken that Kundalini energy for spiritual growth. In fact, you generate a flow of energy that allows for expansion in all areas of your life.

IMPROVES ATHLETIC PERFORMANCE

Trainers in all kinds of sports have long advocated abstaining from sex before a sporting event. Like many others, they feel that engaging in sex, and more specifically ejaculating, weakens your performance. As we've seen, there are a number of nutrients in sperm, and by expelling them and expending energy, you weaken your body for a while following ejaculation.

Many athletes say that they feel more powerful, alert and focused when they don't engage in any kind of sexual activity before an event. That results in a better performance on the field. Muhammed Ali and Mike Tyson are two well-known, successful athletes who made it their practice to abstain from sex prior to a fight.

MAKES YOU HAPPIER

Many people feel guilty following masturbation, and the expenditure of energy can bring them down as well. This is particularly true for those who have become addicted to the habit. The physical reasons behind this are related to the repeated stimulation of the pleasure-seeking centers in the brain. Essentially, they become overstimulated, which reduces the sensation of pleasure due to decreased dopamine levels. Abstaining from masturbation and ejaculation means your dopamine levels stay in the normal range, and you stay happier as a result.

GIVES YOU MORE TIME FOR OTHER THINGS

If you remember being a teenage boy, you know how much of your time can be taken up with masturbation and thoughts of sexual desire. This might still be the case for you even though you're a grown man.

If you're engaging in masturbation and excessive sexual activity, you know that it takes a lot of your time. That's time you could be spending on other activities that can enhance your professional career as well as your spiritual growth and personal life in areas unrelated to your sexual desires. Just think about all the things you could get done if you cut out excessive sexual activity.

A CASE STUDY ON THE BENEFITS

There's nothing like hearing someone talk about their personal experience to illustrate the benefits of semen retention. Jenson is a 32-year-old man from Germany who works in the financial field. He is a regular contributor to an online forum on semen retention and has kindly allowed me to share his story.

Jenson was in his early 20s when he started noticing how his excessive sexual activities were draining his vitality. He noted that he felt as though he was "drying up". Being an avid reader, he began to learn about how to integrate his love life with his spiritual life without completely suppressing his sexual activity. He did not want to be celibate.

He began to study Tantric and Taoist practices around sexual cultivation. He was heartened to learn that he wouldn't have to stop having sex, just stop overindulging in it.

He also was interested in how abstaining from overindulgence would help to deepen his relationship with his partner. He learned that he could have sex without ejaculation, and in that way, he could cultivate the sexual energy, circulate it to share it with his partner, and then store it within his own body. That helped him decide that he needed to try this for himself.

At first, it was difficult for him to go for 30 days without ejaculating, which was the first test he set for himself. But when he finally managed to do it, he noticed that his energy levels improved significantly. In fact, he said the difference was "like night and day". Before practicing semen retention, he needed several cups of coffee to help him get up and become fully alert in the morning. He said he literally had to drag himself out of bed on some days.

After 30 days of practicing semen retention, he found his energy levels were soaring. He also needed less sleep. This makes sense because your body puts a lot of energy into semen production. It pulls resources and nutrients from your organs and other body structures to incorporate into replenishing semen. It redirects your body's energy that normally focuses on cellular repair and self-maintenance.

When you're no longer in a constant state of a semen deficit, your body can focus on other processes, and that means you experience a boost in your energy levels.

Along with his increased levels of energy, Jenson also experienced a significant improvement in his focus. Previously, he had trouble focusing on one thing at a time, and his attention jumped from one subject to the next. He was, as he described himself, "scatterbrained".

After practicing semen retention for 30 days, however, he was able to maintain his focus on his creative passion, music. He was able to stay focused on a task until he finished it. With semen retention, he could now use the zinc that was normally used for semen production to help his brain function better. This not only meant a better focus but a better memory as well. He noted the brain fog he had sometimes suffered from previously was gone.

Another benefit that Jenson experienced was a boost in motivation. He found he had so much energy that he wanted to stay busy. He was studying more, improving his skills, increasing his creative output, going to the gym, and getting everything done that he needed to do. He noted that he had never had that kind of energy before in his life. He called it "incredible", something that made him feel "like Superman".

He also experienced a boost in confidence. In his teenage years, Jenson had low self-esteem, a result of acne after puberty, and it lasted into his 20s. He was a shy individual who could barely bring himself to talk to women. He had suffered from this for a long time, but everything changed when he began practicing semen retention. He could feel himself radiating confidence. He became "comfortable in his own skin". He attributes this to the fact that he was no longer being depleted of the masculine energy he needed to feel confident in his manliness. He notes that prior to this experience, he felt like he had an "empty tank", but after practicing semen retention, he felt full and energised. His vital energy was up, and he not only felt great physically, he felt great about himself, which is the root of all positive actions.

Semen is, after all, the source of masculine energy, and conserving it made him feel powerful for once in his life. Because he was feeling that way about himself, he was also radiating that newfound confidence and masculinity outwards, which made him much more attractive to women. Even though he had a partner, he noticed a subtle shift in attention when he was around women. He sensed they were more interested in him and could sense his "aura" of masculinity.

Each time you ejaculate, your body produces prolactin, a hormone that inhibits testosterone levels and is part of what makes you feel so listless after ejaculating. Since he wasn't ejaculating, his body wasn't producing as much prolactin and his testosterone levels normalized after a long period of deficiency.

By practicing semen retention, Jenson was radiating masculine energy and, of course, women noticed. Further into his journey with semen retention, he found that women began to approach him, something that had never happened to him before. He also found his own desire was increased. But now he could more easily channel that into other activities in his life, such as his work and his desire for success in the field of music. Additionally, he had a strong desire for personal growth so that he could live his life's purpose.

Jenson noted that the biggest benefit he got out of this practice was "self-mastery". It took intense willpower for him to go the first 30 days without ejaculating, but once he knew he could do that, he realized he could do many other things as well. It was just a matter of self-discipline.

As a result of this momentum, he was able to change other habits that were draining his energy. He stopped smoking marijuana, he stopped getting drunk on weekends, he got his body in shape, and he got his mind in shape by exposing it to inspiring content. In short, he got his life together. While semen retention is not a cure-all, Jenson attributes much of his recent success to the practice.

As Jenson describes it, you can be a man whose sexual desires control him, or you can be a man who controls his sexual desires for a higher purpose. "You can be your own master" is the key message he wants to impart. When you take control of your life in this one way, it can't help but carry over into all other aspects of your life. You can evolve into a devoted, hard-working, balanced and confident man who goes after what he wants. The world definitely needs more of those right now. Semen retention can open the door.

CHAPTER SUMMARY

In this chapter, we have discussed the numerous benefits of semen retention. Specifically, we've discussed the following topics:

- The various benefits of semen retention in all areas of life
- How semen retention works to produce those benefits
- A case study of one young man's experience with semen retention

In the next chapter, we'll discuss the scientific evidence for the health benefits of semen retention.

5

THE SCIENCE BEHIND SEMEN RETENTION

You might be wondering if there is scientific evidence to support the health benefits of semen retention. The answer is yes, and in this chapter we'll look at how these studies were conducted and what they show about semen retention. The scientific studies are referenced and the full details are provided at the end of this book should you wish to read further.

The majority of the scientific research into the benefits of semen retention falls into one of two categories: semen quality and the effects of semen retention on testosterone levels. Let's take a look at what these research investigations have found.

THE EFFECTS OF SEMEN RETENTION ON SEMEN QUALITY

Research into the effects of semen retention on semen quality has included research into the following seminal characteristics:

- Semen volume

- Sperm concentration and total count
- Sperm motility and kinematics (motion)
- Sperm viability
- Sperm morphology (shape and structure)
- Advanced semen traits

Let's take a look at what these investigations found.

SEMEN VOLUME

For semen to be considered healthy, the World Health Organization puts the lowest level of semen volume at 1.5 milliliters per ejaculation. The ejaculate volume is significant since it affects the concentration of sperm.

It was previously suggested that semen volume following abstinence indicated a low semen quality; however, in 23 out of 24 studies conducted on semen volume following abstinence, there was evidence for a considerable increase in semen volume.

The last study didn't find a decline in volume; rather, it found no significant change. Several of these studies also noted higher testosterone levels following prolonged periods of abstinence. The thinking is that it may be the stimulation of higher testosterone levels that is responsible for increased semen volume (Ayad et al., 2018).

SPERM CONCENTRATION & TOTAL COUNT

The concentration of sperm in the ejaculate is measured in millions per milliliter, and it is a critical indicator of semen quality. It is also a prognostic (predictable) factor for the fertility potential of the individual.

Twenty-two studies examined the effect of abstinence on

sperm concentration, and twenty of those studies reported a significant increase in sperm concentration in subjects practicing prolonged periods of abstinence. The greatest increase occurred in the first two to five days of abstinence, but there were still mild increases recorded with longer abstinence periods (those over seven days) (Ayad et al., 2018).

Studies have noted an increase in total sperm count, particularly with the first ejaculation following a period of abstinence. These studies also observed that serum testosterone levels peaked at 145 percent of the baseline level following the seventh day of abstinence. They also found that these elevated levels of testosterone remained constant into prolonged periods of abstinence (Ayad et al., 2018).

SPERM MOTILITY & KINEMATICS

This is an important factor in determining male fertility. The sperm needs to be progressively motile to navigate the harsh environment of the female genital tract and reach the egg. Motility refers not only to the sperm's ability to move but also to generate the driving force necessary to penetrate the egg.

Twelve studies that examined the relationship between abstinence and motility were conducted. Eight of them reported a significant increase in the total number of motile sperm, increasing during the abstinence period. The other four showed no significant difference. Between one and three days of abstinence, the number of motile sperm increased substantially, then that number remained stable between the fourth and seventh day. After the seventh day, there was another increase. After nine to ten days, the number gradually declined (Ayad et al., 2018).

Ten studies investigated the effect of ejaculatory abstinence on progressive motility. Five of these determined a higher percentage of progressively motile sperm in subjects who were abstinent for less than a day. However, there may be some problems with analyzing this characteristic, given that there is a significant potential for counting and interpretation errors created by the misidentification of particulate debris as non-motile sperm. Other studies conducted with better identification methods found no significant difference in motility between the various study subjects (Ayad et al., 2018).

SPERM VIABILITY

This is a characteristic that is routinely examined in a basic semen analysis. DNA fragmentation can dramatically affect sperm viability, and this may be an important indicator of DNA integrity in sperm. Eleven studies examined this characteristic and found no statistically significant association between abstinence and a decline in viability. In fact, the percentage of viable sperm peaked between the second and fifth day of abstinence and remained relatively unchanged. Viability did, however, decline with more prolonged periods of abstinence (Ayad et al., 2018).

SPERM MORPHOLOGY

Sperm has three distinct areas: the head, the midpiece (body) and the tail. Each must conform to stringent criteria in terms of size and shape in order to be considered morphologically normal. Morphology refers to the shape of the sperm.

Research has shown there are problems with DNA integrity if the head is malformed. Additionally, other morphological abnormalities can cause problems with the penetration of the egg. When studying the effect of abstinence on sperm morphology, 14 out of 18 investigations found no association between malformed sperm and increased periods of abstinence (Ayad et al., 2018).

ADVANCED SEMEN TRAITS

Advanced semen traits, such as DNA fragmentation, are analyzed in men who are having problems with infertility despite having a normal semen profile. This analysis assesses the characteristics discussed above. These advanced quality indicators include DNA fragmentation, reactive oxygen species production, seminal plasma antioxidants, and pregnancy rate. Results vary regarding the effects of abstinence on semen quality.

DNA Fragmentation: Of eight studies conducted on this quality indicator, three studies found no significant effect of prolonged abstinence on DNA fragmentation. Four studies, however, found an increase in DNA fragmentation with prolonged periods of abstinence. One study found increased DNA fragmentation after only two hours of abstinence as compared to less DNA fragmentation in the initial ejaculate after three to four days of abstinence. Thus, there are mixed results for this parameter (Ayad et al., 2018).

Reactive Oxygen Species Production (ROS): This is crucial for maintaining vital functions necessary for the sperm to mature. They must remain within normal levels, or the sperm will get into a state of oxidative stress. The studies done on this parameter showed no association between abstinence and the levels of ROS. This comes despite the hypothesis that frequent ejaculation would minimize the adverse effects of ROS (Ayad et al., 2018).

Seminal Plasma Antioxidants: Antioxidants protect sperm against oxidative stress caused by free radicals. One published study was conducted on this parameter, and it found an increase in the antioxidant capacity of seminal plasma after abstinence. Another study in progress has noted that four hours of abstinence leads to significant increases in antioxidant activity. Still, more research needs to be done in this area (Ayad et al., 2018).

The overwhelming evidence of these investigations shows that abstinence either does not affect sperm quality or it is improved, particularly following between three and ten days of abstinence. Moreover, important factors like sperm concentration and semen volume showed large improvements with prolonged periods of abstinence. Additionally, several indicators of sperm quality that had been hypothesized to suffer from abstinence were, instead, not affected by short periods of abstinence.

There are several areas where more research is needed, but the takeaway is that abstinence has a mild to moderate positive effect on sperm quality. Some of this research also found increased testosterone levels, but let's look at some studies specifically designed to measure the effects of abstinence on this crucial male hormone.

ABSTINENCE & TESTOSTERONE LEVELS

There are a number of studies that have examined the effect of abstinence on testosterone levels. One study examined how a period of three weeks of abstinence affected the neuroendocrine response to orgasm induced by masturbation. The study involved ten healthy adult men and measured hormonal and cardiovascular factors. The procedure was conducted twice for each participant before and after the three-week period of abstinence. They had their plasma analyzed for concentrations of cortisol, prolactin, adrenaline, noradrenaline, luteinizing hormone and testosterone concentrations.

The results showed that orgasm increased blood pressure, heart rate, plasma prolactin and catecholamines. That was true before and after the sexual abstinence period. Orgasms did not, however, alter the plasma testosterone levels. What did alter plasma testosterone levels was the period of abstinence. Higher concentrations of testosterone were found following the period of abstinence than what had been the case before. This shows that abstinence does not change the neuroendocrine system's response to orgasm, but it does increase testosterone levels (Exton et al., 2001).

Yet another study examined the relationship between ejaculation and serum testosterone levels. The study was run on 28 participants through two phases. The volunteers were investigated daily for testosterone levels during a period of abstinence. The results showed that testosterone levels fluctuated minimally between the second and fifth days of abstinence. Serum testosterone levels peaked on the seventh day of abstinence. In fact, testosterone levels increased by 145.7 percent over the baseline established prior to the abstinence period. After this peak, there was no regular testosterone fluctuation observed with continuous abstinence (Jiang et al., 2003).

What this study demonstrated was that ejaculation caused variations in serum testosterone levels, which peaked on the seventh day of abstinence. This study was among the first to document periodic changes in serum testosterone levels as well as the correlation between ejaculation and those changes. It also showed the patterns associated with changes in testosterone levels, specifically that the maximum testosterone level is achieved with a minimum of seven days of abstinence (Jiang et al., 2003).

Another study examined the effect of sexual activity on athletic ability, testosterone levels and concentration capacity in 15 high-level male athletes. The participants consisted of eight team players, two weightlifters and five endurance athletes. They completed two maximal graded stress tests on a cycle ergometer as well as a one-hour exercise stress test that was coupled with an arithmetic concentration test. The tests were conducted over two days, with one day including sexual activity and another day without sexual activity. Over the two days, blood samples were obtained for testing the levels of testosterone, and each athlete was monitored using a 24-hour ECG machine (Sztajzel et al., 2000).

The results showed significantly higher heart rates following the stress and concentration tests two hours after engaging in sexual activity. These differences were noted at five minutes and ten minutes after the activities. When the athletes conducted another ten hours after sexual activities, these differences had disappeared. While the athletes' heart rates were higher, they noted no detrimental effect on the maximum workload achieved or mental concentration. The increase in heart rates, however, suggests that an athlete's ability to recover following sexual activity could be affected if he engages in the activity two hours before competition (Sztajzel et al., 2000).

Research has also been conducted on how abstinence might affect pregnancy rates. Several studies have examined the effect of short abstinence periods on pregnancy outcomes. It also measured total motile sperm fluctuations following abstinence. One retrospective analysis found that an ejaculatory abstinence period of three days achieved an 11.27 percent pregnancy rate.

This was the highest rate for pregnancy outcomes even though the total motile sperm count in those individuals was highest following seven days of abstinence. That showed that the total motile sperm count was not predictive of conception, as had been shown in previous studies (Li et al., 2020).

That study contradicted another one done in Mexico, which showed that pregnancy rates were higher in the 4–7 day abstinence period than 1–4 days. That would be more in line with the total motile sperm count.

Authors of yet another study found similar results to the research conducted in Mexico. They found no significant difference in pregnancy rates between 5–7 days of abstinence compared to abstinence periods of 2–4 days. Despite the variable results in these studies, the researchers concluded that there was no significant difference between pregnancy rates in couples practicing short periods of abstinence as opposed to those engaging in longer periods (Li et al., 2020).

The importance of these studies relates to the effects of oxidative stress on sperm storage. The idea was that the longer sperm are stored in the reproductive ducts, the more they would be subject to detrimental effects caused by oxidative stress. That can cause an increase in DNA fragmentation associated with low ejaculatory frequencies. However, the data showed that short abstinence periods alter proteins in a way that actually favors conception. In other words, the fertility potential of sperm is not affected by abstinence, at least over short periods, and can actually improve it. More research is necessary to determine the effects of longer periods of abstinence (Li et al., 2020).

OTHER DOCUMENTED PHYSICAL BENEFITS OF SE-

MEN RETENTION

A study conducted on animals in 2007 found that frequent masturbation lowered androgen receptors in the brain. Androgen receptors are those landing pads we discussed earlier. They are where neurochemicals land when they jump the gap between nerve cells. Androgen receptors specifically help the body to use testosterone. The finding that masturbation lowered the number of these receptors indicates that abstinence from ejaculatory masturbation will help your body use testosterone more efficiently (Phillips-Farfan et al., 2007).

BENEFITS OF INCREASED TESTOSTERONE

One of the most studied and consistently noted benefits of semen retention is an increase in testosterone levels. Even those studies that did not specifically research this aspect noted increased testosterone levels following periods of abstinence. This importance cannot be underestimated as it has widely beneficial effects. Let's take a look at some specific benefits.

The research into the benefits of testosterone began in 1889 after Charles Eduoard Brown-Sequard performed a radical experiment in which he injected himself with liquid extracted from the testicles of dogs and guinea pigs. He injected this liquid ten times over three weeks. Brown-Sequard was a 72-year-old neurologist, and after injecting himself with the seminal fluid from animals, he noted marked physical changes. Specifically, the strength in his forearm flexor increased, he had a more forceful urinary stream, he was more easily able to defecate, and he also noted a subjective improvement in his cognitive abilities. His observations are credited with generating more interest in the substances produced by the testes (Tyagi et al., 2017).

Since that time, testosterone, called the "elixir of life" by Brown-Sequard and his contemporaries, has been studied for its anabolic, metabolic and developmental properties. Early research included numerous androgen (male hormone) studies that examined the problems related to low testosterone levels, notably insomnia, depression, nervousness, impotence and a decreased libido. This has caused experts to debate the use of testosterone replacement therapy in men suffering from declining levels of the male hormone. There are numerous beneficial effects of testosterone on the musculoskeletal system, mental and cognitive health, and in a number of other uses (Tyagi et al., 2017).

Sex hormones play a role in bone growth and its subsequent maintenance in both men and women. Those androgen receptors we discussed earlier play a role in the growth plates in bones and the formation of bone tissue. Testosterone also plays a role in decreasing the resorption of bone and increasing bone mineral density. Testosterone replacement therapy has been used successfully to help men with osteoporosis increase their bone mineral density (Tyagi et al., 2017).

Testosterone is also associated with vitamin D, a vitamin crucial for maintaining bone calcium levels. Testosterone also has a beneficial effect on body fat and lean muscle mass. In a study to measure the effects of testosterone and estradiol (another hormone) on body composition, researchers found that lower levels of testosterone resulted in a decrease of lean muscle mass, strength and size. Moreover, when testosterone was inhibited from being converted to estradiol, the result was an increase in body fat. The study showed the importance of testosterone for increasing muscle mass while decreasing body fat (Tyagi et al., 2017).

In another study, older men who had lower than normal testosterone levels were given testosterone replacement therapy. They experienced improved muscle function and increased lean body mass when combined with strength training. The control group who solely utilized strength training experienced improvements in muscle function, but not lean body mass. The musculoskeletal benefits of testosterone therapy disappeared within six months after discontinuing the therapy (Tyagi et al., 2017).

Studies have also shown that testosterone plays a role in mental health and cognitive ability. One study found that healthy, older men given testosterone intramuscularly demonstrated significant improvements in both spatial and verbal memory. Another two-month study of 51 men with low testosterone levels showed significant improvements in mood as well as a decrease in negative mood parameters, like anger and irritability, following testosterone replacement therapy. It also improved their energy levels (Tyagi et al., 2017).

Studies haven't just been conducted on older men, either. In the first half of the 20th century, studies began into the benefits of testosterone for athletes. When researchers controlled the studies for exercise routines and protein intake — that means they eliminated those factors as possible influences in the study — they found that testosterone accelerated increases in strength, fat-free mass and overall muscle mass in men who exercise. Additionally, young men with low testosterone levels also showed an increase in muscle strength and fat-free mass (Tyagi et al., 2017).

Testosterone is also beneficial for helping with urinary tract symptoms associated with overgrowth of the prostate gland. Older men often suffer from an overgrown prostate gland,

and this constricts the tube through which urine passes — the urethra — so that these men have a weak stream. Because of that, it takes them a long time to empty their bladder completely, and they have to urinate more frequently. In a study of 246 participants given testosterone for one year, researchers found they improved their urine storage capacity and voiding. Several case studies have also shown that testosterone replacement is safe following the removal of the prostate gland as a result of cancer (Tyagi et al., 2017).

Testosterone is also helpful for patients who require rehabilitation. A study of men between the ages of 65 to 90 showed that injections of testosterone were associated with improvements in limb function. Testosterone administration also helps men on bed rest maintain their protein balance, although this benefit was only seen in those patients who could walk daily. The research seems to suggest that the benefits of testosterone administration require physical activity (Tyagi et al., 2017).

While these studies were not testing increased testosterone levels due to semen retention, they show the importance of testosterone in maintaining or improving health in various ways. Since semen retention has been shown to increase testosterone levels, it follows that men who practice it will see some of the benefits associated with higher testosterone levels. These include improvements in muscle strength and mass, as well as improvements in cognitive abilities and a boost in mood.

Taken altogether, the scientific evidence for semen retention suggests numerous physical benefits. Perhaps the most notable benefit is an increase in testosterone levels that can boost mood, improve memory and increase muscle strength and lean body mass. Moreover, a number of semen traits improve, including seminal fluid volume and concentration of sperm. Improvements in the quality of sperm also improves fertility.

So as you can see, there are several documented physical benefits to semen retention, but what about the impact of the practice on your wealth and success? We'll take a look at that in the next chapter.

CHAPTER SUMMARY

In this chapter, we've looked at the scientific studies showing the benefits of semen retention. Specifically, we've discussed the following topics:

- The effects of semen retention on semen quality
- Testosterone levels and semen retention
- Benefits of increased testosterone levels

6

HOW SEMEN RETENTION MAKES YOU MORE SUCCESSFUL

We've mentioned the many benefits of semen retention in previous chapters, but here we want to discuss how some of those benefits actually translate into greater success in all areas of your life.

As we discussed, ancient beliefs describe the process of transmutation of the energy it takes to produce sperm into areas of your life other than procreation. Of course, procreation is a strong instinct in all species, but humans, whose larger brains mean they are more capable of abstract, symbolic thought, have the option to divert the energy put into procreation for other endeavors. It's in the diverting of that energy that they find success. Let's look more closely at what this means.

Men are able to produce sperm once they have reached puberty. The production of that sperm requires a great deal of energy, and that's one reason why, on average, men don't live as long as women. In fact, many believe that the production of sperm to create life also takes a little bit of life away from the man producing it. Thus, by lowering the number of ejaculations you have throughout your lifetime, you will also be able to lower the overall sperm production. This ultimately means you'll live longer, age slower and look better physically. That's one marker of success because it gives you more time to realize your dreams.

We have been discussing how semen retention has been proven to increase testosterone levels, and that alone produces a cascade of effects that help you become more successful in life. First, it is the hormone responsible for masculine traits such as increased muscle mass and better muscle tone. It can also give you more confidence and help reduce symptoms of depression, anxiety and feelings of social awkwardness. In short, it makes you more attractive to prospective partners and more confident in your abilities to be successful. That spurs your creative, innovative and problem-solving abilities to kick into high gear.

As we've also discussed, sperm is full of nutrients that, when conserved, you can apply to other areas of your health and well-being. These include valuable substances that help your brain function better, thereby improving your mental clarity and memory. That works because, after around two weeks of semen retention, your body reabsorbs the sperm, so those nutrients are now recycled to other parts of the body. As a result, you get thicker hair, better skin, brighter eyes, bigger muscles, more facial hair growth and a better functioning brain. You even get a deeper voice. This is the abundant power of transmuted semen energy.

When you practice semen retention, your brain quickly realizes that you are not ejaculating — the mechanism by which life is created. This tells your brain that it has to improve your potential for mating, and that means improving everything about you. This is when you have the opportunity to rechannel your retained energy into creative abilities, willpower, courage and persistence, and these qualities can then be used to accumulate riches in life, create amazing works of art or build the body of your dreams.

Remember that the riches you accumulate in life translate into resources for attracting a mate. Even if you wish to practice absolute celibacy, your brain will still be working behind the scenes to help you find a partner and procreate, by motivating you to improve yourself. That's because millions of years of evolution shaped your anatomy, brain and motivations, and fine-tuned them for reproduction. But you can choose how to use those motivations and your new-found energy. But when you do, the results are often incredible.

The underlying action of your brain to help you attract a partner is essentially an irresistible force, and when you're being guided subconsciously by this force, you'll find you have fierce motivation, drive and ability to spring into action. The key to applying that ability to other areas of your life is control over your sexual energy. For example, by willfully directing that energy into your business pursuits, you'll develop mental clarity and acuity that will bring you great success in any professional endeavor.

One scientific study examined why, traditionally, most men don't really begin to succeed until they are in their 40s or 50s. It found that when they were younger, they tended to dissipate their energies through sexual indulgence, and that kept them from realizing their full potential. When they got into their 40s and 50s, they began to focus less on sexual pursuits and more on other areas of their life. As a result, they achieved the success that had eluded them formerly. But don't take my word for it. Let's look at some testimonials from successful men in different professions about the power of refocusing sexual energy.

DAVID HAYE: FORMER WORLD HEAVYWEIGHT CHAMPION

David Haye likened semen retention to a lion who hasn't eaten anything for a while. That makes him one dangerous animal. Haye stated that he doesn't release for six weeks before a fight. He doesn't have sex or masturbate; no ejaculation. By the time the fight rolls around, he's got a lot of pent-up energy that's ready to be released, and he releases it in the ring on his opponent. Similar strategies also worked for Mike Tyson and Muhammad Ali. Both of them went years without releasing any semen, and there's no arguing with their success.

SARVESH SHASHI: A 28-YEAR-OLD WORTH $15 MILLION

Sarvesh is a rare man, indeed. He is a consultant in the wellness industry whose clients include Jennifer Lopez, Dwayne 'The Rock' Johnson and Naomi Campbell. And, believe it or not, he's a virgin. When he was growing up, he says he was arrogant and aggressive. He originally wanted to be a cricket player. He got into yoga because his father felt it would help him with the sport by controlling his emotions.

His yoga teacher taught him how to calm himself and took away his anger and ego. He asked Sarvesh to live by five precepts that included celibacy and semen retention, and Sarvesh followed his advice to the letter. While he doesn't believe there's anything harmful about having sex or masturbating, he abstains as part of his own journey towards self-actalization. He believes it helps him to be "clean from within".

When asked how abstinence changed his life, he credited his ability to channel the creative energy found in semen to his brain through meditation and celibacy. He noted that his self-discipline took away the distractions that had plagued him earlier in his life. That allowed him to focus on his goals. The way he looks at it, ejaculating produces a few moments of pleasure, but by abstaining, he has created true sustainable pleasure through spiritual and professional success.

STEVE JOBS: CO-FOUNDER OF APPLE
Unfortunately, Steve Jobs is no longer with us, but he was the genius behind Apple, and he also practiced semen retention. He wasn't celibate, but he did refuse to reach orgasm and ejaculate, except when he wanted to have children. He firmly believed in conserving his seminal energy for his work. Toward that end, he practiced tantric sex to help him harness that intense energy. The work he did revolutionized the world through computer technologies, and of course, he was a billionaire many times over.

Here's a few historical figures known to have practiced semen retention:

WINSTON CHURCHILL: PRIME MINISTER OF THE UK
Winston Churchill is widely considered to be one of the best leaders in history. He helped defeat Adolf Hitler, and he practiced semen retention. He once remarked that he was able to write so much because "I don't waste my essence in bed."

That likely played a big role in his extraordinary achievements.

MICHELANGELO: SCULPTOR & ARTIST
Michelangelo is arguably the most gifted artist in history. He was able to create remarkable sculptures, including "David" and "Pieta", both of which are held as treasures for all humanity. Michelangelo was also a brilliant painter and an architect — clearly, an overachiever. He planned St. Peter's Basilica, and he painted the ceiling of the Sistine Chapel. He is also known to have abstained from both sex and masturbation. His contemporary biographer, Ascanio Condivi, wrote about his monk-like chastity, and this is supported by the fact that in many of his works women are depicted as manly in form. By abstaining from sex, he was able to focus on creating those amazing works of art.

NIKOLA TESLA: INVENTOR & FUTURIST
Nikola Tesla is commonly known as the man who invented the 20th century. He was known to be celibate for his entire life. He redirected that energy into his professional life, and it has brought us some of the greatest achievements at a scale that has yet to be repeated.

In the early 20th century, he invented a way to transmit electricity wirelessly, and he created devices that caused earthquakes and manifested ball lightning. He was a handsome, successful man who, had he not rejected aristocratic money for his inventions, would have been the first billionaire in history.

All the same, he made a conscious decision to reject sexual pleasures. He stated in an interview that women were the greatest thieves of energy, and therefore, of one's spiritual power. He went on to say that he decided to preserve that energy for himself so that he could create what he wanted.

LEONARDO DA VINCI: THE ARCHETYPE OF RENAISSANCE MAN

Leonardo Da Vinci is one of the most renowned men in history. He was an expert in many diverse pursuits: art, engineering, human physiology and much, much more. He had a grand ambition to be a master of all trades, and he most certainly achieved that. He was also a lifelong bachelor, and there is no indication he ever had an interest in romantic relationships or sexual acts. Nothing in his diaries or works indicated otherwise.

However, he did speak about it when he said that the procreative act was so disgusting that it would surely die out if it had not become a human tradition and if there were no "sensuous dispositions and pretty faces". From those comments, it is clear he practiced semen retention, and the redirection of that energy produced phenomenal works for all humankind.

SIGMUND FREUD: NOTED PSYCHOLOGIST

While Sigmund Freud is a controversial personality, there's no disputing his influence in the field of psychology. His theories have polarized the world, and interestingly, they all center around sex. He came up with the famous Oedipus complex that states boys desire their mothers and come to see their fathers as competition. That's why there's such friction between father and son. He also believed women had "penis envy".

He thought masturbation resulted in anxiety, and he also believed that sexual activity was incompatible with the achievement of great works. He did have a wife, but after he turned 40, he became fully celibate until his death. Despite his discredited theories, he is still considered the Father of Psychoanalysis. That's a legacy that cannot be ignored, and it is likely his choice to become celibate that helped him achieve his goals.

NAPOLEON HILL: AMERICAN SELF-HELP AUTHOR

Napoleon Hill is best known for his book, *Think and Grow Rich*. It is rated as among the top ten best selling self-help books of all time. His books all talk about how to achieve success in life, and he devoted an entire chapter in *Think and Grow Rich* to semen retention and diverting sexual energy into other areas of your life. He wrote that sexual transmutation is a vital first step for anyone who wants to become rich.

As you can see by now, many famous, successful men have used the power of sexual transmutation to achieve their goals. Let's look at some specific reasons that abstinence can create success.

INCREASES CORE STRENGTH

If you're an athlete, probably the number one thing you need is core strength. Core muscles are active when you're withstanding opposing forces like gravity, and they impart strength to all parts of your body. Without strong core muscles, you're likely to suffer from a number of injuries, and although exercise is a great way to strengthen your core muscles, ejaculation depletes them of strength. If that happens, it will destabilize your body and prevent other muscles from reaching their maximum potential strength. That's why the athletes on the list above know (or knew) they had to retain the energy from their semen to increase their physical power. The longer they practiced ejaculatory abstinence, the more explosively powerful they had the potential to be in their sport.

IMPROVES ROMANTIC RELATIONSHIPS

There's perhaps nothing that can cloud your judgment more than sex. When you remove that from the equation, you can see your romantic partner for who they really are, and you can determine if you genuinely enjoy their company. Sex won't be distracting you from your problems. Instead, you'll have to find real solutions or decide to discontinue the relationship. In short, abstinence will save you a lot of time and heartache as you work to establish a solid, long-term relationship with someone you love. Moreover, what occurs when you have sex with someone is a spiritual exchange that has important implications for your entire life. Practicing ejaculatory abstinence helps you focus on your partner's pleasure and on building a life together.

IMPROVES DISCIPLINE

Bucking a strong natural desire requires discipline. You have to manage not only your sex life but other areas as well. As you learn to control your actions, you strengthen your mind and your ability to focus on what is important in your life. Lust without wisdom often results in damaged relationships, unplanned children, prison, divorce, depression and countless other problems. It requires discipline to contain that kind of lust, but when you're able to stick to a standard that you set yourself, you'll find you're able to develop the kind of self-discipline that brings success to every area of your life.

HEIGHTENS CREATIVITY

When you harness sexual energy, you are able to convert it into a powerful tool for improving your life. Your imagination becomes much more vivid as your awareness increases. You're motivated to pursue various other goals to expend that pent-up energy, and your physical stamina gives you the ability to do just that.

Because of the connection between your brain and your libido, you're hard-wired to go to extreme lengths to satisfy your sexual desire; however, when you channel that same energy and apply it to other goals, your life can become completely transformed. You'll be able to conceptualize the life you want to live, create ideas to bring it into reality, and finally live the dream life you've always wanted. You're using a powerful natural energy that's responsible for all life on Earth. By becoming aware of that energy and harnessing it, you can "birth" your many other goals into existence.

SPIRITUAL GROWTH
As we have already discussed, numerous spiritual traditions teach that sexual energy is part of a complex field that relates to your spiritual energy. When you awaken the feminine Kundalini energy sleeping in your root chakra, it rises through the other chakras until it unites with masculine energy at the crown chakra. When that happens, you experience the universal oneness that is your natural state. You awaken into the reality of your own divinity. It doesn't matter whether you embrace this literally or as a metaphor to achieving your version of spirituality through your enhanced ability to focus on what is important in your life and the values you believe in. Redirecting this sexual energy into aspects of your spiritual life allows you to experience a much more vivid sense of the divine.

The main thing to understand about sexual energy is that it is a powerful creative energy. It's not evil, but when it's not controlled, it can be destructive. By refraining from overindulgence or practicing outright abstinence, you use that creative energy to maximize your potential in every area of your life. You can generate success in your professional life and build deep, loving, long-lasting personal relationships. You can grow personally, professionally and spiritually. Sexual energy is analogous to crude oil in that it is valuable, powerful and an important resource, but to maximize its power, you have to refine it. Only then can you use its power to fuel productive and constructive creation in your life.

In the next chapter, you will learn about NoFap and semen retention.

CHAPTER SUMMARY
In this chapter we have discussed the numerous ways in which semen retention can help you be more successful. Specifically, we've covered the following topics:

- How sexual energy is transmuted into energy to use in other parts of your life.
- Numerous famous, successful men who have utilized the practice of semen retention to achieve their goals.
- The reasons why it works in various areas of your life.

7

NOFAP AND SEMEN RETENTION

If you've done any research into semen retention, you've probably run into the word NoFap, and you might be wondering if NoFap and semen retention are the same thing. The answer is that they are not, but they are related. Let's look at what is different and exactly how they are related.

NOFAP
NoFap emerged out of an online conversation that started in 2011 between people who had given up masturbation. The term, which is now in fact a trademarked name and business, is derived from the slang term "fap," which is internet lingo for masturbating. It comes from the sound that you make when you're engaging in self-pleasure — fapfapfapfap.

NoFap began as a discussion forum, but it soon became a website and organization that doesn't just promote quitting masturbation, but also abstaining from watching pornography as well as other kinds of sexual behaviors. The target audience is primarily straight men, but it is open to all genders and sexual identifications.

BENEFITS OF NOFAP

Many of the benefits are similar to what you get with semen retention, and for the same reasons. For example, because you are no longer engaging in sexual behavior or ejaculating as frequently as before, men practicing NoFap also experience an increase in testosterone levels and more motivation to improve their life. The benefits include:

- It boosts your self-confidence
- You feel happier
- You experience more motivation and stronger willpower
- You experience lower levels of anxiety and stress
- It heightens your spiritual experience
- You experience more self-acceptance
- You experience a better attitude towards, and greater appreciation for, the opposite sex

There are also similar physical benefits to what you experience with semen retention. These include higher energy levels; greater muscle growth; better sleep; improved mental clarity, concentration and focus; increased stamina and better overall physical performance; improvement in, and sometimes even a cure for, erectile dysfunction; and improved quality of sperm. As we've already discussed, many of these physical benefits and some of the mental benefits are related to increased levels of testosterone, and these have been demonstrated in clinical studies.

NOFAP AND PORNOGRAPHY

One of the differences between semen retention and NoFap is that NoFap doesn't completely prohibit ejaculating; rather, proponents believe that you should give up masturbating and viewing pornography. That has a similar effect as semen retention, given that you're not engaging in sexual activity resulting in ejaculation as much as you would be otherwise. But when you're with a partner and have sex, they don't necessarily advocate for a dry orgasm. They are happy for you to release within the context of a relationship. Whereas with semen retention, you are not ejaculating in order to reap the many benefits. NoFappers are primarily focusing on what the Taoists would call overindulgence.

Concerning pornography, NoFap recommends giving it up due to the negative effects it can have on your sex life, your attitudes towards sexual partners, and your life in general. They also argue that by watching pornography and masturbating frequently, you waste time as well as energy in destructive activities. You also develop obsessive and unhealthy attitudes and beliefs about sex. In fact, in the largest ever survey within the NoFap community, they found the following effects on men who watched porn and masturbated frequently:

- Their desire for a steady mate declined, and only those who were able to find different mates frequently were able to maintain arousal. This is something called the Coolidge Effect. It's a tendency toward novelty-seeking behavior, and this is precisely what porn trains viewers to do.
- Only 20 percent of people who regularly watched porn felt they were able to control their sexual desires. That means 80 percent felt they could not control their desires.
- At least 32 percent of those surveyed reported they watched five or more hours of internet porn each week, and 59 percent said they watched between four and fifteen hours

each week.
- Approximately 50 percent of those surveyed were virgins. Their only sexual experience came from masturbation.
- Among college-age males, some 42 percent visit porn sites regularly.
- More than half — 53 percent — developed their porn habit between the ages of 12 and 14. Another 16 percent started watching porn before they were 12.
- Two-thirds (64 percent) reported that their tastes in porn became more extreme and deviant.
- Among those surveyed who were aged between 27 and 31, 19 percent suffered from premature ejaculation, 31 percent had difficulty reaching orgasm, 25 percent were disinterested in sex with their partner, and 34 percent had problems with erectile dysfunction.
- Once they committed to ditching their masturbation and porn habits, 60 percent felt their sexual function had improved.
- Among that same group who committed to no masturbation or porn, 67 percent experienced a self-reported increase in energy levels.

You can see that there's certainly enough evidence to suggest that porn can negatively impact your life. It's also easy to see how much time pornography and masturbation can eat up when you're in the grip of an addiction. Imagine having that time to apply to other areas of your life.

While semen retention and NoFap are not the same exact things, they clearly share several benefits. Semen retention differs from NoFap in that NoFap doesn't advocate avoiding ejaculation; rather, it simply argues that by giving up the overindulgence in sexual activities represented by porn and masturbation, you can gain better control over your life and experience the benefits of at least short periods of abstinence.

Of course, as we've discussed, semen retention is all about ejaculatory abstinence. You might achieve that through complete celibacy for a period — what NoFappers would call "hard mode"— or you can achieve it through the dry orgasm, whereby you experience an orgasm but don't ejaculate.

You might be thinking that it's kind of old-fashioned to be against masturbation, and while that is true, there are also benefits to be had from abstaining from it. Let's look at a few points you may not have considered before.

SOCIAL OR SPIRITUAL PRESSURE

Many people feel like masturbation is a sin, and many religions argue it is. Because many individuals believe that masturbation is immoral, there is also a stigma attached to it. If you want to understand that, think about some famous people who have been caught masturbating. There's something a little seedy about them, and many people think they're immoral as a result.

Because of the social and religious stigma attached to masturbation, a number of myths have developed designed to produce anxiety and fear in those who dare to masturbate. You've likely heard you'll go blind, but maybe you haven't heard that it can cause you to grow hair on your hands. These, of course, are completely false, but still, these rumors persist.

Because those kinds of rumors still circulate, particularly among teenagers, many people experience negative feelings of shame, guilt and even self-loathing when they masturbate. For that reason, it's important to distinguish between choosing to abstain from masturbation and ejaculation for the benefits we've discussed rather than feeling as though you have to because of religious or social stigmas attached to the behavior. You shouldn't feel guilty if you masturbate, but choosing not to can produce several benefits.

UNDERLYING CONDITIONS MAKE IT DIFFICULT

Some people might have health problems that make masturbation difficult for them. It can be a frustrating experience, for example, if you have erectile dysfunction, low libido, or something like post-orgasmic illness syndrome where you become ill immediately following ejaculation. Masturbation can also be difficult or upsetting if you have been traumatized sexually.

MASTURBATION CAN BE ADDICTIVE

Anything in excess is not going to be good for your health, and that's just as true for masturbation as it is for drugs or alcohol. A good rule of thumb is that if what you're doing is interfering with your life, you've got a problem. As we've discussed, masturbation becomes addictive because it triggers the brain's pleasure centers in the same way drugs and other addictive substances do. You can tell that you might have a problem if you experience the following regarding your masturbation habits:

- You feel frustrated if you can't do it whenever you like
- You can't concentrate on much of anything else
- You do it to the point you injure yourself
- You suffer from symptoms like premature ejaculation or erectile dysfunction
- It's affecting your sexual relationship with your partner

NOFAP HARD MODE

NoFap has a more strict version that advocates abstaining from ejaculation, which is similar to semen retention, but it also says you should completely give up porn. It has some specific rules, and these are good rules for anyone who is practicing semen retention, whether they class themselves as NoFappers or not. The rules include the following:

- No porn allowed. This is good for keeping you from becoming sexually stimulated. If you're practicing semen retention, it's helpful to avoid exposing yourself to porn.
- No erotic images of any kind allowed. For the same reason as above, avoiding all erotic imagery will help to keep you from becoming stimulated to the point where you might not be able to control your urgues.
- No masturbation, even without porn. While it is possible for you to orgasm without ejaculation, it takes a great deal of muscular control, and if you're masturbating a lot, it's going to be more difficult for you to achieve that.
- No orgasm. Again, it's possible to have a dry orgasm, but it's not easy, so it's better to avoid orgasms in this case.
- No sex. This is particularly true if you are just getting into semen retention. Of course, you may also choose celibacy, but if you want to have sexual relations with an intimate partner, you should avoid sex until you feel you have adequate control over your orgasms.
- No lusting. Lust leads to impulsive behavior, and that's generally not conducive to semen retention or NoFapping.
- Follow these rules for at least 90 days. Once you have control over your sexual desires and behaviors, then you can choose to resume some degree of sexual activity.

Hard mode is definitely a difficult choice for someone who is just starting out, but it's necessary to gain control over your sexual behaviors. It depends on your level of addiction to sex and masturbation, but for many people, hard mode is a definite must. It will help you build a good foundation for mastering your own desires, and it helps you gain the benefits of either NoFap or semen retention much faster than if you continue to engage in sexual activities sporadically. If you are uncertain about whether it's right for you, ask yourself the following questions:

- Is porn, masturbation or other kinds of sexual activity stopping me from achieving my life goals?
- Have I accomplished my life goals for the age I have reached?
- Do I even know what my life goals are?
- Do I have the will-power to engage in sexual activity without ejaculating?

If the answers to those questions give you pause, then it's likely you'll want to pursue hard mode to gain more control over your life and begin to focus on achieving those things you deem most important. If you do choose to practice hard mode, you must follow the rules for at least 90 days. After that, you can continue in an easier mode. For example, you might have or wish to have an intimate relationship with a partner. After the 90 days, you can resume that relationship, but it's important to remember that you want to genuinely treasure your sexual experiences and your partner as well. The idea is to break any shallow, addictive behavior associated with your sexual experiences.

When you follow hard mode, you'll experience a number of

benefits as a result. You'll gain those benefits many times faster than if you were still engaged in sexual activity or thoughts, and you'll find you're taking the achievement of your dreams in life more seriously. You'll gain enormous energy, meaning you will be ready to rise and shine even before the alarm goes off. Of course, your testosterone levels will soar, and potential partners will notice. You'll also gain all those great benefits of increased testosterone levels, like more muscle mass and a happier disposition,

It's important to remember that while we are naturally driven to reproduce, and that means having sex, you can take that enormous energy source and use it to do other things as well. In fact, overindulging in sex makes your sex life worse, as we've seen. If, on the other hand, you start conserving your sexual energy, you'll be able to channel it toward achieving great things.

HOW TO REACH 90 DAYS IN HARD MODE

I know it's a hard sell to swear off any kind of sexual activity or even thoughts for 90 days, but let's look at a strategy you can use to achieve that goal. You can even go longer using these tactics.

The first thing to do is break that 90 days down into smaller chunks. That makes the overall goal seem easier to achieve and gives you different ideas for redirecting your energy. Let's look at three phases for achieving 90 days of no sexual activity, desires or thoughts.

PHASE 1: 0 - 30 DAYS

This is probably the most important phase, precisely because it's the most difficult. It's possible you may relapse during this phase, but just keep following the strategies described here, and you'll get there.

USE PARENTAL MODE

If you want to avoid lustful thoughts, you need to stop yourself being exposed to stimulating images or situations. On your computer, use parental mode to block any pornographic sites. If that won't work for you, ask a friend to change the password to unblock those sites. That way, you won't be able to access the parental control mode to change it once it is set to block porn. There are a number of software programs you can use for this, but one good one is called Covenant Eyes. It completely blocks all porn sites, and it also makes you accountable to someone else. That's a strong motivator to reach your goal.

CHANGE YOUR ENVIRONMENT

It's easy to have a lot of stimulating materials in your environment, so we need to clear that out. That means removing sexy posters on the walls, sexually stimulating books, sex toys and sex magazines. It's also important to try to get yourself out of the house more and socialize, or even just go for a walk. If you're just staying alone in your house or room, it's easy to start fantasizing. If you must stay in, try opening the windows to make your room or house feel less isolated. Put up motivational posters on the wall, and turn on the lights. It also helps to change up your routines as this disrupts your habit triggers. For example, if you're accustomed to coming home from work and engaging in self-pleasure on the couch, arriving home from work has become your trigger to engage in the habit of masturbation. If you disrupt the trigger by doing something like going for a walk or heading straight to the gym after arriving home, then you're breaking that cycle.

TRY JOURNALING
This can help you express your feelings, but it's important not to write an erotic novel here. Instead, focus on defining your goals, writing about why doing this is important, and discussing what you intend to do with your new-found energy. You might be rolling your eyes at the idea of keeping a journal, but you will be surprised at how much this technique can help you achieve your goals. It's a great habit.

EXERCISE
Exercise can put you in a good mood since it releases endorphins — the body's feel-good hormones — and it will keep you occupied and keep your mind off sexual activities. As a bonus, it will also get you into great shape.

PHASE 2: 30 - 60 DAYS
By the time you're in this phase, you're doing pretty good. It's difficult to even reach ten days in hard mode, so take a moment to congratulate yourself if you've made it this far. By this point, you have less of a chance for a relapse, but you still can't relax. You've got to keep up all of the things you were doing in Phase 1, but now we'll add a little purpose to your journey. This means identifying what it is you want to do with your life.

It's easy to let sexual pursuits distract you from your life's purpose. It's also important to identify what that purpose is so you can focus your sexual energy on achieving it. If you don't do this, then you will likely experience a relapse.

When you are identifying your life purpose, you want to be clear and specific about it so that you have a well-defined reason for abstaining from sexual pleasure. How do you do that?

1. Think about things you love doing and identify any that can be turned into a career.
2. Think about those things you find easy to do. Are there possible career paths there?
3. It's a cliche, but it's a valuable question — if money wasn't an issue for you, what would you do with your time?

Once you've determined what you feel is your life's purpose, write it down. Write it out clearly and specifically. If your goal is to become a millionaire, be specific about how much money you want to earn. If your goal is to become an artist, determine what kind of artist you want to be, how much money you want to make, and how famous you want to be. It's in this specificity that you start to put your brain to work on the subconscious level to achieve what you've set as a goal.

Next, write out a plan for how you will go about achieving your life's purpose. What do you need to make it a reality? Do you need more education or training of some kind? Do you need to get certain materials? Whatever you need to do to make this your lived reality, write it down. The steps you need to take will be milestones to achieve on your way to your broader goal. And when you achieve them, celebrate that accomplishment.

At this point, determine a timeline for accomplishing these goals. Be sure to give yourself enough time for each milestone because if you don't, you're setting yourself up for failure. So be realistic.

Once you've defined your overall goals and your milestones to achieving them, set up daily, weekly, monthly, and even yearly planning meetings with yourself.

In your daily meetings, begin by reading your goal out loud and planning what steps you will take that day to get closer to your next milestone. In the weekly meeting, you can plan the following week's milestones, celebrate what you achieved in the previous week, and adjust your timeline for any milestones you could not achieve. In your monthly meetings, you examine what you achieved and make adjustments for the following month, and in the yearly meetings, you have a broader overview of what you have achieved and any adjustments you need to make. You're treating your dreams like you would a project you're managing for a company. That will keep you accountable and on track.

During this phase, you also want to replace habits like masturbation and pornography. It's important to have something to do that relaxes you as long as it isn't something sexually stimulating. Develop an exercise plan, take up painting, read a good book, or hang out with some friends. Take time to enjoy your life and smell the roses. In fact, it's likely you're just now noticing the roses after quitting sex for this long! So, really take them in with your whole being.

PHASE 3: 60 - 90 DAYS
This is the last phase, and if you've made it this far, it will be the easiest phase. That doesn't mean, however, that it will be problem-free. This is where you need to get back into socializing and back into your life. You're going to do it without the goal of having sex, but instead, you'll want to focus on your friends and family in a way that you might not have been doing for some time. Really get to know and understand them.

If you don't have anyone close to you, go out and make

some new friends. It's easy to isolate yourself when you've been overindulging in sexual pleasures, particularly those like masturbation and pornography. That's why it's important to go out and start living your life again. However, you need to avoid putting yourself in situations where you're going to feel like having sex. You're not going out to pick up a partner, but to really focus on your friends and family. If you're with a partner, really get to know them at a deeper level. Let yourself see them as the complex human being they are instead of as a form of sexual release for you. Doing that will take any relationship you have to a much deeper level.

Hard mode is difficult, and you don't have to do it for your entire life, but you *can* do it for 90 days. It builds a foundation upon which you can gain control over your sexual behaviors, and that will help you start living your life with more clarity and purpose. It's about deciding what's important to you and how you really want to live your life. Do you want to live it in spurts of five minutes of pleasure? Or do you want real, engaging, long-lasting and deeper relationships and achievements? The choice is yours.

CHAPTER SUMMARY
In this chapter, we've discussed the similarities and differences between NoFap and semen retention. Specifically, we've discussed the following topics:

- What is NoFap?
- How is NoFap different from semen retention?
- Some new perspectives on masturbation
- What is NoFap hard mode, and how can it help with semen

retention

In the next chapter, you will learn some detailed techniques for sex without ejaculation.

8

SEX WITHOUT EJACULATION

If you've decided you want to practice semen retention, but you still want to have sex, then this is where you'll learn the specific techniques. Of course, one of the choices is to abstain from sex altogether, but this may not be something you want to do, particularly if you're in an intimate relationship with a partner.

It is still possible to practice semen retention even if you have sex. As discussed in the previous chapter, ideally you want to try to abstain from all sexual activity during the first 90 days of a semen retention or NoFap commitment. After that period, you can resume sexual activity. The idea is, as the ancient wisdom advises, to avoid overindulging.

There are a number of techniques we'll cover that you can use to have sex without ejaculating. You'll need to learn the basics of controlling your muscles to avoid ejaculatory orgasm, but once you've mastered that, you can apply it while engaging in some profound sexual techniques that will undoubtedly thrill your partner and deepen your relationship. First, let's look at the basics of muscle control.

HOW TO AVOID EJACULATION

The first step is to locate the muscles of your pelvic floor. Try to stop urinating midstream or prevent yourself from passing gas. Notice which muscles come into play when you're doing that. Those are the muscles of your pelvic floor. They are called Kegel muscles, and you'll want to exercise them. You can do that in any position — standing, sitting or even while walking or lying down. You simply contract those muscles. Again, think about preventing yourself from passing gas or stopping urination midstream. The key is that you ONLY want to contract your Kegel muscles. You should keep your butt, thighs and abdomen relaxed, and you should be breathing freely. You should do ten sets of contractions at least three times a day to build up your muscle control.

Next, you need to learn to control these muscles during sex of any kind. You'll want to relax any tension you have in your jaw, butt and legs. Relax your pelvis as well and avoid allowing energy to build up excessively in that region.

As the orgasm approaches take long, deep breaths. You might even hold perfectly still for a few moments to calm your body. During that time, you can put your attention on your partner. As an orgasm approaches, and you have come to the point of no return, squeeze those pelvic floor muscles just like you do with your Kegel exercises, open your eyes and stop any stroking or thrusting. This will result in a dry orgasm. You'll achieve the pleasure of orgasm without ejaculation.

Another technique is to apply pressure to the area between your scrotum and your anus. This causes a retrograde ejaculation where the seminal fluid goes into the bladder instead of out of the penis. But the retrograde orgasm is not the best way to keep that positive energy flowing. You'll have to practice these techniques to get them just right, but when you do, you can move on to some wonderful kinds of sexual experiences.

TANTRIC SEX
Tantric sex is all about connection, whether it's with yourself or your partner. The word is derived from ancient Sanskrit, and it means "to weave energy". The Hindu Tantras were all about enlightenment, and as we discussed in an earlier chapter, they focused on spirituality more so than the Taoist traditions. Tantric sex is something that transcends the sexual and spiritual planes. It's a deeply meditative, intimate experience, one that truly weaves your energy with that of your partner.

As with yoga, Tantra is about both physical and spiritual awareness. You become more in-tune with your body and what gives it pleasure, as well as the way it feels that pleasure. When you pay attention to what your body wants and needs, you're better able to make sure that you're fulfilled, and you're better able to understand what will fulfill your partner as well. It's all about getting to know your body, your partner's body and the energetic flow of joy between them. When you do this, both you and your partner will experience intense satisfaction, even without ejaculation.

How do you practice Tantric sex? Here are some practical tips you can use to implement this technique.

PREPARE YOUR MIND
Remember that this technique is a spiritual practice, and the goal is to make a deeper connection with your partner. Your mind here is just as important as your body, and you want to feel that connection between the two of you in a spiritual way. You want to unite the mind, body and soul. You also need to be

willing to step out of your comfort zone. For that reason, it can help to spend 10-15 minutes in gentle, meditative breathing before you begin the tantra practice. This will allow you to look inward and examine your thoughts. There are other daily practices that will help you keep your mental processes in the right place for this practice. Here are some techniques to get you in the right frame of mind:

MEDITATION

- Sit in a quiet, comfortable, but alert position. You don't want to fall asleep.
- Focus on your breath and breathe all the way down into your lower back and belly. You'll want to breathe this way for 15-30 minutes.
- As you're breathing, you want to get in touch with your mind. What are you thinking? Are you stressed? Are you concerned about fulfilling your desires? Just notice what your thoughts are and how your body responds to them.

STRETCHING

- Stretch for at least a few minutes each day.
- Gently stretch each limb. Let yourself feel the muscles as they release tension.
- Notice your thoughts, particularly those that might be weighing you down. As you stretch, release not only the tension in your muscles but the tension in your mind.

JOURNALING

- Spend at least 10 minutes each day writing in your journal.
- Let your writing flow freely, as you notice which thoughts are blocking your growth.
- When those thoughts arise, write them down. Then, examine them carefully.
- Challenge those negative thoughts that are blocking your growth. Are they really true? The chances are they reflect old wounds that need to heal. Explore where these came from and then commit to replacing them with positive thoughts. For example, if you have negative thoughts about your self-worth, replace those with, "I am worthy of love and success." As you make these replacements and begin to dwell on them, you retrain your brain to be more optimistic.

This kind of self-healing process is critical for getting in the right frame of mind to practice the self-control necessary for both Tantric sex and semen retention. But that's only part of the equation. You also have to prepare your space.

PREPARE YOUR ENVIRONMENT

Tantra is a holistic experience, one that's not just about arriving at the destination of an orgasm, with or without ejaculation. It's about the journey you undertake to get there. That's why you need to arrange your environment in such a way as to encourage a positive, relaxed mindset so that you can enjoy that journey, whether it's one you make with a partner or by yourself. Here are a few ways to prepare your space so that you will enjoy the total experience.

- **Temperature**: You want the room to be at a comfortable temperature. Adjust the thermostat at least an hour before your practice so that the room temperature is just where you want it to be. This is different for each person, but remember that you will likely be undressed, so keep it at a temperature where you will not feel either too hot or too cold.
- **Mood**: You want to set a calm, romantic mood. That can be done with candles or tinted light bulbs. Candlelight adds romance to almost any space, while soft, red bulbs can add a sensual touch. You might also like to add rose petals or other romantic items to enhance the sensual feel.
- **Scent**: You want each of your senses to experience the romantic mood you're setting. Scented candles, hanging flowers, essential oils or incense sticks can all create a pleasant smell that helps you feel sensual without being overwhelming.
- **Softness**: You want to feel as though your space is "soft" and welcoming. You can accomplish this with touches like satin blankets or plush cushions. You could create it with a plush throw rug or something that feels soft to the skin.
- **Romantic Vibe**: Create a sensual vibe that will appeal to you and your partner. This can be accomplished with some slow music, something you and your partner can move to sensually.

Once you've set up your space, it's time to think about building the moment. Let's look at the options.

BUILDING THE MOMENT TOGETHER
You also want to build the moment when engaging in sensual

play with a partner. It doesn't have to always end in sex either, but whether or not it does, here are some tips for implementing Tantric principles into those moments you can share.

FOREPLAY
Foreplay can take many forms. It can be a massage, a shower together, or even whispering those sweet nothings. The form really doesn't matter as much as being fully present for the experience. That's true for both partners. Here's a technique to do that:

- Sit facing your partner and look into one another's eyes.
- Breathe deeply and feel appreciation for them being in your life.
- After five minutes, begin to touch each other in a sensual manner. Take turns massaging each other's legs, arms, neck and other parts.
- After another five minutes, begin to kiss each other. Stick to just kissing as you continue to experience every physical sensation fully.

You might begin foreplay in other ways, but don't jump right into the act of sex. Move more slowly, take it one step at a time, and be sure to both explore and experience each sensation.

THE SEXUAL EXPERIENCE
Your goal as a couple doesn't have to be sex; it might be just about making a deep connection. That's the really important part, in any case. If you do opt for sex, take it slow and get creative. Use new positions, touch each other in different ways, or explore new desires. The important thing is to immerse

yourself fully in the experience as you let the tension build. When you get near to orgasm, you can engage the muscle control techniques discussed earlier to prevent ejaculation. Of course, a Tantric sexual experience with your partner doesn't have to end in sex.

TOGETHERNESS WITHOUT SEX

You can also have some extremely profound sensual experiences with your partner without having sex. You can use these techniques to draw you closer together and enhance your intimacy even when you're choosing to remain celibate. They can also make for powerful yoga techniques for practicing on your own.

1. **Cuddling**: Lying down with your partner allows the two of you to weave your energies together and nurture a deeper connection. A spooning position is a great one for sending energy to your partner. The person at the back will be sending energy, and the one in front will be receiving it. Harmonize your breathing so the energy can flow freely between you.
2. **Yab-yum or Lotus**: You can do this energy technique with your partner or by yourself. If you do it with a partner, sit cross-legged while they sit on your upper thighs and cross their ankles behind your back. Stare into each other's eyes and breathe in sync. If doing this by yourself, sit cross-legged with your back straight and place your palms on your knees. Breathe slowly and deeply.
3. **Hand on Heart**: Sit cross-legged facing your partner and place your right hand on their heart. Have them place their right hand on your heart. Close your eyes and tune into

your partner's physical rhythm. Focus on the emotion and energy of their body. Let the connection build between your partner's heart and your hand, as well as between your heart and their hand. If you're by yourself, sit cross-legged with your back straight. Place your right hand on your heart. Close your eyes and tune into your heart's physical rhythm as you focus on the emotion and energy. Let the connection build.

4. **The Relaxed Arch**: Have your partner sit upright on the bed or floor with their legs straight out in front of them. Sit on your knees across your partner's lap. When you're comfortable, slowly begin to arch your back until you can rest your head between your partner's legs as you grab hold of their ankles or feet. To do this by yourself, sit on your knees and arch your back until you can rest your head on the floor or bed. Stretch your arms around your head with your palms up.

ORGASM CONTROL

Orgasm control is a crucial element of Tantric sex, and of course, it's also vital for semen retention. As you edge closer to an orgasm, you want to pull yourself back from climax and instead let the tingling, orgasmic sensations move through your body. Once the sensation passes, slowly begin to build the tension again. Repeat this cycle over and over again until you reach an explosive orgasm. When you do, contract the muscles as we've discussed to avoid ejaculation. You can experience a dry orgasm as many as five times, so let yourself fully enjoy the sensations you're experiencing.

A FEW THINGS TO REMEMBER

There are a few things to remember when practicing Tantric sex. These will enhance your practice and bring you a truly unique experience.

1. **Being naked is optional**. You might start out clothed or remove them all. It's also sensual to remove one another's clothes slowly.
2. **Focus on your breathing**. Each of the techniques we've discussed places great importance on deep breathing as part of Tantra. This helps keep you in the present moment and allows you to immerse yourself fully in the experience.
3. **Engage all of your senses**. You want each of your senses immersed in this experience. You want to feel sensual softness, hear sexy music, see each other's eyes, smell enticing aromas and savor the taste of your partner's body. Engage all of your senses and fully experience each moment.
4. **Go slow**. It's vital not to rush the experience. You want to create a profound, sensual experience, and that means taking your time. Relax your mind, and be present for each experience.
5. **Explore.** This refers to fully experiencing every part of your partner's body. Stroke them slowly, use your tongues to explore one another's mouths, and let yourself experience the warmth of their body next to yours.
6. **Experiment**. Try new things and think outside the box. Don't be afraid to explore one another's fantasies and have fun as you do. It will make the experience more intense, and you'll be looking forward to the next opportunity to be together.

Tantric sex is one way to slowly, sensually experience love with a partner, and it's a great adjunct to semen retention. But it's not the only way to incorporate semen retention into your intimate, sexual experiences.

KAREZZA TECHNIQUE

Some men may want to avoid orgasm altogether, particularly if they find it difficult to control ejaculation. If that's your situation, this technique is just what you're looking for. The word Kerezza comes from the Italian word for "caress." The technique involves touching, stroking, fondling, gazing and even penetration; in short, everything but orgasm and ejaculation. Too often, people have sex like rabbits when they should make it more like a tortoise.

The Karezza method was first described in 1931, but even so, not a lot of people are familiar with the name. Like Tantric sex, it typically improves intimacy, closeness and communication between you and your partner. That's because the practice is less physiological and more spiritual. Moreover, you strengthen the connection with your partner with this technique, in part because, like Tantric sex, you're engaging more of your senses while remaining present. As with any sexual experience, there are a few tips that can make the experience more sensual, intimate and intense.

1. **Choose your partner carefully.** This is not a technique you want to choose for a one-night stand. You want to have someone you can trust, and you want someone who values intimacy.
2. **Discuss why.** It's important to be on the same page regarding why you want to use this technique. This is

particularly true if both of you have different reasons for using it.
3. **Establish the ground rules.** You need to make sure you both know what the rules are. For example, are there parts of your body that you don't want to be touched? Will you caress each other for a particular amount of time, or is there a word you will use to indicate you're ready to calm down? What should you each do if you feel you're going to orgasm? These are all questions you should talk about with your partner. It's important that both of you lay out your expectations since orgasm for you is not among them, and penetration is optional.
4. **Determine the timeline.** Karezza can go on for hours, but it doesn't have to; in fact, some people will just do ten minutes of it and then stop, completely satisfied.
5. **Debrief.** It's also important to talk about what you experienced after. If there was something your partner did that felt especially good, let them know. Also, if you didn't like something, discuss that so you can change it up the next time.

The idea behind karezza is to create a close union, one in which each act creates a reconnection of sorts between the two partners. Toward that end, as with Tantric sex, there are a few tips to keep the union fully satisfying.

MINDSET

You want your mindset to be one of mental and spiritual wholeness. Use meditative techniques to get your mindset right. Explore your own values and share them with your partner. You want your mindset to be positive, warm and caring. Part of that relates to thinking more about love than passion, so you can convert your passion for sex into a passion from the heart. Also, it helps to be sensitive and alive to your partner's tones, smells and touches. When you emphasize love and affection, you can put your focus on that as you keep your orgasm under control.

TIME AND SPACE
Since you both have to be on the same page, choose a time when you can both be alone without feeling hurried or like you might be interrupted. You also want to make sure you're comfortable with pleasant surroundings and a warm temperature, just like you did for the Tantric practice.

NO FOREPLAY
Because you're experiencing intimacy without orgasm, foreplay doesn't work well for this technique. You don't want to build sexual tension with the goal of an orgasm. The goal here is mutual adoration and a generous touch. You want to bond with your partner and increase your intimacy. Instead of foreplay, you want to get into bed together and lie in a comfortable position while you gently caress and hold one another. Structure this part of your experience, so you have a better chance of changing those old habits around traditional sex.

WHAT IF YOU FEEL LIKE YOU'RE LOSING CONTROL?
If you begin to feel as though you might be closing in on orgasm while making love, pull yourself back into a relaxed feeling using deeper, longer breaths that come from your abdomen. That will reverse the increased muscle tension and tendency

to restrict your breathing, both of which come with orgasm.

SLOW SEX
You want to start the sexual experience in a position that doesn't allow much movement so that you won't slip back into familiar habits. You want to move slowly, and even sometimes, remain completely still. It's in the stillness that magical and extremely gratifying experiences can result. This technique means the lovemaking will happen in waves as erections come and go. Be sure to communicate the sounds of pleasure and touch when you feel them. You might even fall asleep while you're still inside your partner, but that's okay because waking up will be that much more enjoyable.

Because this practice is not goal-oriented, it can instead activate your relaxation response. Normal sex stimulates the body's fight or flight (sympathetic nervous system) response because you're essentially doing what you need to do to survive biologically. You're passing on your genes, or at least, that's what your body thinks. That type of sex produces powerful orgasms, but not profound feelings. Bonding behaviors like karezza signal to the body that it's safe. That stimulates bonding and relaxation. The kind of bonding that comes from this practice will leave you with a feeling of connection that's truly deep and lasting.

BEST POSITIONS
Because you don't want to slip into the mode of traditional sex, it's important to avoid those positions that will stimulate those old habits. For that reason, it's important not to penetrate too deeply, particularly when you're just starting out. You want to be open, fully relaxed and still as your body gets used to being

inside your partner without wanting to ejaculate and thrust hard.

It's helpful to avoid the missionary position since that typically triggers the mating/ejaculation urge. Different positions, such as your partner on top, is fine, but make sure you both move slowly. Side to side motion is good. You can explore other positions as well. Really, any position works as long as you can stay relaxed.

It's important to remember that karezza doesn't necessarily produce rapid results, but the effects are cumulative. You want to practice it for at least three weeks before you can really compare it to traditional sex. You'll likely find yourself with an enhanced sense of joy and optimism as well as connectedness towards your partner. That's a state of being in the flow. The overall effect of karezza is a re-creation of the intensity and love of the honeymoon period of your relationship, and it produces a lighthearted kind of energy between you and your partner.

You can see that these techniques for avoiding orgasm can produce an intense bonding experience for you and your partner. These are some great ways to avoid ejaculation while still intensely enjoying the sensual experience.

CHAPTER SUMMARY
In this chapter, we've discussed techniques to enjoy sex without ejaculation. Specifically, we've talked about the following topics:

- How to physically prevent ejaculation
- Tantric sex — how it's practiced and why
- Karezza technique — how to practice it and the bond it

creates

In the next chapter, we'll discuss techniques to cool down sexual tension.

9

FASTING, MEDITATION, COLD SHOWERS AND MORE

If you are committed to semen retention, and particularly if you've chosen to be celibate for a short time, you're going to need to find a way to control your sexual urges. Better yet, you want to redirect that energy into other, more productive areas of your life. You might be wondering what you can do to keep yourself from thinking about one of the strongest urges known to us.

There are a number of techniques and practices that can help you with this and, in the process, lead you towards becoming the best version of yourself. Take a look at the list below and see which ones resonate with you in particular. They can make for powerful tools as you embark upon your new journey.

SELF-AWARENESS
Getting to know yourself is a good way to keep your mind off sex. Becoming more aware of what you like and don't like and how you affect the other people in your life gives you something to focus on. Additionally, many people don't know why they

are triggered sexually, and this is a good time to figure it out. Once you know more about yourself, you'll understand what triggers your powerful urges. Moreover, if you have had any traumatic experiences in your life, those things that remind you of that past can trigger a need to seek out comfort, which often takes the form of sex or self-pleasure. When you become more aware of what triggers your urges and why, you become more adept at disarming them.

INTERPRET YOUR FEELINGS WITH WORDS
Sometimes, feelings of vulnerability and fear can cause you to seek out something to deflect those emotions. Often, what you seek out is something sexual or detrimental to your health, such as junk food or spending excessive time playing video games. When you actually name your feelings, you can more readily identify your fears and subsequent needs, and when you identify your needs, you can find a more appropriate way to fulfill them. If you can't name your feelings, you can't name your needs, and you'll be unable to meet them. Once you're able to name and meet your needs, you won't automatically seek out sex to make you feel something different. So when you're feeling triggered, write down exactly what you're feeling and what need or pattern of thought links you to that feeling. For example, you might be feeling apprehensive, and the need associated with that is to be comforted, or you might be feeling bored, and the need associated with that is to be stimulated. Once you understand that you need some kind of deflection, you can now choose other things aside from sex to meet your needs.

SET YOUR THOUGHTS ASIDE

When you're feeling those sexual urges, briefly acknowledge them, but then set them aside for the moment. You're not rejecting or suppressing them; this might make you feel guilty or ashamed. In this way, you can validate your thoughts and needs but wait to explore them. That can help them fade into the background and allow you to refocus your attention on something else.

TAKE A BREAK
It's easy for your thoughts to wander when you're tired or bored. When you give yourself a break, you can lower your urges. Taking a walk or having a healthy snack can recharge your energy reserves and take your mind off sexual thoughts. It also positively affects your emotional mindset by allowing you to reset your thinking and get back on track with productive pursuits.

WRITE IT DOWN
If you simply can't get your mind off those sexual urges, then you can find a different way to get them out of your system. Try writing them down in detail. Of course, you'll want to make sure you're in a place where you cannot act on any sexual urges. You also should take a little time and do this. You can even save what you've written for a time when you can explore those urges more intimately. For example, maybe you're fantasizing about your partner. Preserve your fantasy by writing about it. When you're being intimate together, even if it's without sex, you can discuss what you've written as you bond with each other.

PLAY SOME MUSIC

Music can be a way to distract yourself from your thoughts. If you put on something that makes you want to dance, it can help tone down your libido and warm up your body.

PHONE A FRIEND
It can also help if you've got someone to talk to about your feelings, particularly if you know someone who's also practicing semen retention. It's kind of like getting a sponsor for addictive behavior. Like the sponsor, someone who understands what you're going through can give you some tips as well as empathize with what you're feeling. They can also remind you of all the positive reasons why you're doing this. Moreover, sometimes what's triggering your sexual urges is nothing more than a desire for closeness, and a good friend can often fill that need while also helping you get your libido under control.

DISTRACT YOURSELF
There are a number of things you can do to distract yourself from sexual urges. It helps to get outside where you can't fulfill those urges. Go for a walk, meet some friends for dinner or a drink, read a good book outdoors, go bowling, or do a fun activity. When you make a change in what you're doing, you'll notice how quickly your thoughts change.

EXERCISE
Get out and get your body moving. Even if what you're looking for is comfort, exercise causes your body to release endorphins, and as a result, you'll start feeling better. Exercise also keeps your body moving and gives you more energy to get done the tasks that will move you forward with your goals.

TRY FASTING

Whether you're doing it for religious reasons, for weight loss, or as part of a healthy lifestyle, fasting decreases certain hormones. These, in turn, can impact your sexual desire. One study of people fasting as part of Ramadan found drops in the serum follicle-stimulating hormone (FSH) as well as in sexual desire, body weight and the frequency of sexual intercourse. The researchers concluded that intermittent fasting might be associated with decreased sexual desire among participants (Talib et al., 2015). It makes sense because fasting tells your body that you're not getting enough food, and as a result, your body starts focusing on staying alive rather than reproduction.

COLD SHOWERS

A cold shower does a number of things. First, it stimulates the parasympathetic nervous system. Remember the sympathetic nervous system? That's the fight or flight nervous system. It's what gets stimulated when you're sexually aroused. The parasympathetic nervous system is the opposite of the sympathetic nervous system. It's your "chill and relax" nervous system, and it's turned on by the vagus nerve. Cold showers stimulate the vagus nerve, which turns on the parasympathetic nervous system, and that helps you calm down. It's something to do anytime you're feeling aroused and has been tested down the ages as a way of bringing down sexual urges.

MEDITATION

Meditation is a great way to train your mind, redirect your thoughts and understand your emotions. You can get to know yourself better this way too, and it helps your brain to form new, positive habits. Aside from redirecting your thoughts, meditation helps you to dampen your sexual urges by grounding you in the present moment. It's also a great way to better understand your life purpose, and it has numerous physical benefits, including lowering blood pressure, reducing anxiety and preventing depression. It's one good habit you'll be happy to have in your tool kit for life.

GET CREATIVE
Remember sexual transmutation? This is when you can really get into doing just that. When you're feeling those sexual urges and not sure you can control them, get creative. Sit down and paint, sculpt, play music, write creatively or do something else creative. As you start to channel that energy into something creative, you'll see that hobby will really take off. It might even become part of your life purpose. You could even use that creativity to make plans for something you want to do to change your life or solve a problem you've been having trouble with recently.

FILL UP YOUR SCHEDULE
Everyone needs time to relax, but when you've got time on your hands, it's easy for those racy thoughts to come calling. While you need to leave yourself some downtime, try to keep your schedule as full as possible. This will keep you active and keep your mind busy. Additionally, sex is often an answer to boredom, so if you keep yourself occupied, you won't feel bored. The less time you give yourself to think those sexy thoughts, the more successful you'll be at controlling the urges.

THINK OF THE LEAST SEXY THINGS YOU CAN
Think of things that will turn you off. Perhaps, it's nails on a

chalkboard, a break in a sewage line, car horns, an ambulance siren, or whatever it takes to turn you off. Put those images in your mind when lustful thoughts come calling, and you're likely to forget all about the sexual imagery. It's kind of like the mental equivalent to taking a cold shower. This is something, however, that you can only use occasionally, as the power of it diminishes over time. Still, it can be very effective in those situations where you need to stop yourself from thinking sexual thoughts right there and then.

CHANGE YOUR DIET

Some foods act as an aphrodisiac to increase your sexual desires, so to stop being horny, you might need to adjust your diet. Since ancient times, people have understood that certain foods increase your libido, but you might not know that there are also "anaphrodisiac", which are foods that lower your sex drive. Asparagus, watermelon, almonds, oysters, figs, chili peppers and strawberries are all foods that are likely to increase your sex drive. Alcohol also can put you in the mood, particularly wine. So, to reduce your libido, you might want to cut down on alcohol and avoid these stimulating foods.

Also, to know what's triggering your libido specifically, it can be helpful to keep track of your meals and compare your sexual energy level with the food you've consumed. You'll soon identify those foods that are increasing your sexual desire, and you can then avoid then.

Soy-based foods, foods that are high in saturated fats, vegetable oil, salt and sugar can surpress your sex drive the most. However, these foods are also unhealthy so it's not a good idea to begin consuming them in abundance. Instead, here are some foods that can lower your sex while ensuring you still stay healthy: mint, flaxseed products, beets and cruciferous vegetables. Granted, these are not the most exciting food choices, but they do the job.

SAMPLE DAILY SCHEDULE

It can help to see an example of how you might structure your day to prevent yourself from being distracted by sexual thoughts. It entails keeping yourself busy but also taking some downtime that is focused on something other than sexual desire. Here's an example that might help you to structure your days so you'll have success when practicing semen retention and/or NoFap.

- **6:00 AM**: Get up early and start the day with 30 minutes of meditation.
- **6:30 AM**: Follow your meditation with 30 minutes of journal writing. Try writing about your life's purpose, the goals you must hit to achieve that purpose, and your timeline for achieving those goals.
- **7:00 AM**: 30 minutes of exercise.
- **7:30 AM**: Eat a healthy breakfast.
- **8:00 AM**: Self-hygiene — shower, shave, brush your teeth and get dressed.
- **9:00 AM - 5:00 PM**: Work.
- **5:00 PM**: Catch happy hour with a friend.
- **7:00 PM**: Eat a healthy dinner.
- **8:00 PM**: Spend 30 minutes reading something inspiring. This could be something related to your professional goals, your spiritual goals or just general knowledge or an inspiring biography.
- **8:30 PM**: Spend some time on a creative hobby. Write a

short story, paint a picture or make some pottery; really anything creative.
- **9:00 PM**: Watch the early evening news.
- **9:30 PM**: Engage in your evening meditation practice.
- **10:00 PM**: Early to bed, early to rise!

Of course, this might not match up perfectly with your schedule, and you should adjust it accordingly, but it gives you an idea of how you can fill up your day with things that keep you active as well as activities that help relax you. You have some social time as well as alone time, and you engage in self-reflective activities to keep you growing personally.

CHAPTER SUMMARY

In this chapter, we've discussed activities and ideas that can help you control your sexual desire while you're practicing semen retention and/or NoFap. Specifically, we've discussed the following topics:

- Various ideas for lowering your sex drive
- Some techniques for sexual transmutation
- A sample schedule for keeping busy and keeping your mind off sex

In the next chapter, you will learn of any potential drawbacks of semen retention.

10

ARE THERE ANY DOWNSIDES TO SEMEN RETENTION?

You might be wondering if there are any risks associated with practicing semen retention. You also might have heard people say it is dangerous but don't know if that's true. Let's take a look at some of the claims that have been made about this practice to see what's true and what's not.

CLAIM: FREQUENT EJACULATION PREVENTS PROSTATE CANCER

One of the most commonly reported risks associated with semen retention is that you need to ejaculate frequently to prevent prostate cancer. The claim is that by ejaculating more, you clear out "old semen" that has been found to be associated with prostate cancer. Additionally, you lower your testosterone levels, and that helps prevent prostate cancer since it's associated with high levels of the male hormone.

    This is based on the claims of one study conducted in 2016 that hasn't been replicated. In fact, other studies were not able to find the same connection between ejaculation and lowered risk of prostate cancer. One study even showed that younger men who masturbated more often actually had a slightly higher risk of developing prostate cancer (Shambo, 2020).

What's more, a big problem with the 2016 study is that the researchers couldn't determine if it was a situation of causation or correlation. Perhaps men who masturbate more are also more likely to engage in certain other habits. It could be that one of those other habits that is responsible for reducing prostate cancer risk, instead of the frequent ejaculation.

The contradictory reports coupled with the lack of a causal relationship in the 2016 study indicate there's no scientific consensus on the subject of semen retention, frequent ejaculation and prostate cancer (Shambo, 2020).

Another problem is that there haven't been any scientific studies on men who practice semen retention when it comes to prostate cancer. Nor any studies on men who practice non-ejaculation in a healthy manner by engaging in Tantric sex or karezza and live a healthy lifestyle. It's likely that diet, energy management and exercise all play a larger role in prostate health than how frequently you ejaculate. Additionally, it's not necessarily the orgasm with ejaculation that may prevent prostate cancer; it could be the stimulation of the prostate itself. As we've seen, the two things needn't go together (Shambo, 2020).

Additionally, while some studies have claimed that men at the low end of ejaculation frequency are more likely to die prematurely, those who claim this are not allowing for the problems these men may have that caused their low ejaculation frequency to begin with. For example, a man may not be engaging in frequent sexual activity, including ejaculation, because they are sick or engaging in other unhealthy habits that stifle their sex drive. Thus, there is no causal relationship between ejaculation frequency and premature death cited in these studies (Shambo, 2020).

One of the claims is that retaining semen causes stagnation of sperm, which then damages the prostate gland. The problem is in a healthy male, the body reabsorbs the retained semen and converts it into energy for other areas of your life. It doesn't result in the stagnation and congestion claimed by those who argue it causes prostate damage. The tendency of disregarding other lifestyle factors is a significant problem from a scientific perspective.

CLAIM: SEMEN RETENTION IS A SEXUAL DISORDER

This is a particularly interesting claim given that no one has studied the long-term benefits or risks of lovemaking without ejaculation. In fact, science has shown relatively little interest in the subject of ejaculation and male orgasms. Should a man choose not to ejaculate, this is technically classed as a sexual disorder in medical terms.

That's despite the fact that thousands of years of Tantric and Taoist traditions have demonstrated the health benefits of the practice of semen retention. This speaks to a larger problem within western medicine — separating the mind from the body and both from the spirit. The refusal of western medicine to understand the connection between the three or even to acknowledge that a connection exists has resulted in the dismissal of thousands of years of Eastern philosophies with demonstrated efficacy. Furthermore, the labeling of semen retention as a disorder has resulted in significant social stigma.

Anyone affected by a stigma of any kind can suffer social consequences such as ostracization, loss of friendships and bullying. Men who engage in semen retention may be the subject of gossip, and of course, anything related to sex tends to fuel even more rumors. If it is believed such men have a sexual disorder, as semen retention is called, then they can face extreme social judgment. People often react to their gut fears before listening to rational explanations. This can have many negative consequences. So what can you do?

Perhaps the best option when practicing semen retention is to tell no-one, apart from your partner if you have one, as it will affect them. The next best thing that men who are practicing semen retention can do is to try to educate their friends and family regarding exactly what it is and what it is not. It is not a sexual disorder. It is an ancient practice that has many health benefits. It is not perversion; in fact, it is the opposite. You are controlling your desires and redirecting that energy to other areas of your life. The proof will be in the pudding. When you are the best version of you, your family and friends will see the benefits for themselves. They'll see your success and your boundless energy. That will help them understand that what you're doing is not a disorder.

CLAIM: TOO MUCH DESTRUCTIVE ENERGY

Some people claim that men who practice semen retention suffer from too much restless, and potentially dangerous, energy. This couldn't be further from the truth, as long as you're channeling that energy into other areas of your life using the techniques we've discussed. It's the very principle of semen transmutation. You're taking the energy found in your semen and directing it to other parts of your life where you're putting it to use to find success.

Instead of masturbating, you're engaging in creative activities like painting or writing. Instead of having sex, you're planning your next business move. You're not holding onto that energy; you're expending it on other activities that will bring you professional, personal and spiritual success.

The truth is that there are no scientifically (or otherwise) demonstrated risks associated with semen retention. This is a choice you're making for yourself, one you're doing to become more spiritually, professionally and physically healthy, to become the best version of you.

The benefits of semen retention have been demonstrated for thousands of years, and you can use them for the same reasons the ancient Taoists did. You can find spiritual contentment, professional achievement, and profound intimacy with a romantic partner. When people see the change in you, all thoughts of a social stigma or sexual disorder will fall away. They'll likely want to know what your secret is.

CHAPTER SUMMARY

In this chapter, we've discussed the purported drawbacks of semen retention. Specifically, we've covered the following topics:

- The purported risks of prostate cancer
- The idea that semen retention is a sexual disorder
- The purported risk of having too much energy

In the next chapter we will present some final thoughts.

11

CALL TO ACTION

Semen retention is an ancient tradition associated with the use, manipulation and circulation of energy. Sexual energy is a prime driver in all species, including humans. The subconscious desire to successfully mate is behind virtually everything we do. It's a powerful source of creative energy. Alternative and traditional practitioners have recognized it as such for thousands of years.

Ancient Tao and Tantric texts have touted the powers of avoiding overindulgence with regards to sexual energy. They have noted that we can use this powerful resource to fuel our professional, creative, personal and spiritual pursuits with astounding success. All energy is cyclical. It cycles through our bodies and connects us to one another. Sexual energy is a creative force that has significant power to modify our behaviors and actions for the better. If you can harness this powerful energy source, you can direct it to any area of your life that you desire to improve.

It works so well because of the numerous physiological benefits that seminal energy provides. It feeds your brain with phosphorus and zinc, and that fuels your creativity. It also helps you think with more clarity and improves problem-solving skills. It raises your testosterone, and that gives you energy. It builds muscles, gives you confidence and improves your appeal to potential partners. It also encourages the kind of calculated risk-taking that many business people have used to build empires.

You can decondition yourself as a man, regardless of your age or background, from being a slave to your sexual desire. You can gain control over your sexual nature and make a conscious choice as to what to do with that energy. That simple fact is liberating. You don't have to be a slave to your primal instincts any longer. You can build confidence by gaining control over one of your most powerful natural drives.

When you gain the confidence and ability to control your own desires, you'll see numerous positive changes in your relationships, marriage and attitude towards sexuality. You'll fill that void you've always sensed but couldn't quite put your finger on. You will truly be free. That's what this book is really about: helping you find the freedom to soar.

By taking this journey, it's really a loving attitude you are showing yourself. You're choosing to take control over that wild dragon inside you. When you find yourself riding the dragon, you'll become confident in your ability to conquer anything in your life. You'll know you can achieve success and live your ideal life. You have the power within you.

You can use semen retention to become the best you, and the best you is a powerful, creative, intelligent and spiritual being. Start taking control today by implementing the practices described in this book. When you start on your journey, you'll soon realize that you can achieve anything that you focus your new-found energy on. Tap the abundant power within you and become who you were always meant to be.

In that spirit, I now throw down the gauntlet to you. I ask you to simply complete phase 1 of the 90-day challenge — 30 days of semen retention — using the techniques outlined in this book. After 30 days assess honestly how you feel, your energy levels, your body composition, your motivation and how other people relate to you. I'm betting you will be blown away by what semen retention can do and you'll be encouraged to make it a fixture of your lifestyle.

Try the 30-day challenge and open the door to the new you!

Wishing courage and clarity on your life's journey,
J. Peterson

12

REFERENCES

A. (2020a, August 16). *7 Masculine Benefits Of Semen... Forever Alpha*.

Ames, H. (2020, September 25). *What to know about semen retention. MedicalNewsToday*.

Antonyan, C. (2019, August 14). *What Is Female Ejaculation? – Where Does The Liquid Come From?*

Ayad, B. M., Horst, G. V., & Plessis, S. (2018). Revisiting The Relationship between The Ejaculatory Abstinence Period and Semen Characteristics. *International journal of fertility & sterility*, 11(4), 238–246. https://doi.org/10.22074/ijfs.2018.5192

Bailey, A. (2020, September 24). *What is Tantric sex? How to enjoy Tantric sex with your partner. GoodtoKnow*.

Banihani, S. A. (2017). Vitamin B12 and Semen Quality. *Biomolecules*, 7(4), 42. https://doi.org/10.3390/biom7020042

Bedard, M. (2016, June 6). Magic Fire Semen. Gnostic Warrior By Moe Bedard. https://gnosticwarrior.com/magic-fire-semen.html

BROJO. (n.d.). Learn about semen retention - BROJO. Retrieved October 31, 2020.

Bui, K. (2020, June 5). How To Practice Sperm Retention. You Be Relentless.

Christian, S. (2017, August 9). 10 Reasons Why You Should Quit Watching Porn.

Cirino, E. (2018, March 7). How Does Karezza Work? Healthline.

Cohen, B. (2019, October 13). 4 Supernatural Benefits of Practicing Abstinence. - Bryant Cohen.

Cruz, M. (2020, August 30). How Semen Retention has changed my life. Bossless Mindset.

Exton, M. S., Krger, T. H. C., Bursch, N., Haake, P., Knapp, W., Schedlowski, M., & Hartmann, U. (2001b). Endocrine response to masturbation-induced orgasm in healthy men following a 3-week sexual abstinence. World Journal of Urology, 19(5), 377–382.

Ferguson, S. (2020, January 28). Does Masturbation Have Positive or Negative Effects on the Brain? Healthline.

Henderson, R. (2020, August 21). Semen retention: how to orgasm without ejaculation.

James, B. (2020, May 31). *Why Semen Retention Is The Key To Your Success & Competitive Edge In Life.*

Jeffrey, S. (2020, July 8). *Sexual Transmutation: A Definitive Guide to Sexual Energy.* Scott Jeffrey.

Jiang, M., Jiang, X., Zou, Q., & Shen, J.-. (2003). *A research on the relationship between ejaculation and serum testosterone level in men. Journal of Zhejiang University-SCIENCE A, 4(2).*

Joshi, S. (2020, July 21). *How Staying Away From Sex and Masturbation Helped Me Become a Millionaire.*

June, S. (2020, October 13). *How To Stop Being Horny: 10 Effective Ways To Control Your Sexual Urge.*

Kassel, G. (2020, May 21). *How to Have Multiple Orgasms — Because Yes, It's Possible!*

Kooner, R. (2016, December 2). *Vitamin A increases male fertility/ Human-Fertility.Com.*

Li, J., Shi, Q., Li, X., Guo, J., Zhang, L., Quan, Y., Ma, M., & Yang, Y. (2020). *The Effect of Male Sexual Abstinence Periods on the Clinical Outcomes of Fresh Embryo Transfer Cycles Following Assisted Reproductive Technology: A Meta-Analysis. American Journal of Men's Health, 14(4), 155798832093375.* https://-doi.org/10.1177/1557988320933758

Liwanag, R. (2018, October 4). *The 6 Foods That Could Absolutely Kill Your Sex Drive.*

Lybrate. (2016, February 17). Advantages And Disadvantages Of Masturbation - By Dr. Rushali Angchekar. https://www.lybrate.com/topic/advantages-and-disadvantages-of-masturbation/caa37a45e6317bb1572a64010f11a991

M. (2020b, October 26). NoFap Hard Mode: Gain All the NoFap Benefits 10x Faster!

Mangay, P. T. (2016, September 23). 6 Powerful Ways to Stop Being Horny: No Masturbating or Sex. LovePanky - Your Guide to Better Love and Relationships.

Miller, A. M. (2018, May 21). Karezza Is The Orgasm-Free Way To Improve Your Sex Life.

Mindbodygreen. (2020, February 24). Let's Talk About Semen Retention, Tantra's Best-Kept Secret For Male Pleasure.

Moral Revolution. (2015, May 13). How Do You Manage Your Sex Drive Without....You Know?

MSI College. (n.d.). The Benefits Of Sperm Retention. Gye! Retrieved October 31, 2020, from https://guardyoureyes.com/articles/tips-suggestions/item/the-benefits-of-sperm-retention

Müller, A. (2020, June 3). Kundalini Energy: What It Is and How to Awaken It Within You.

NoFap. (n.d.-a). BENEFITS OF SEMEN RETENTION. NoFap®. Retrieved October 31, 2020.

NoFap. (n.d.-b). Sexual Transmutation as First Step to Riches. NoFap®. Retrieved October 31, 2020.

Owusu, K. (2020, March 25). Semen Retention Benefits: Using Your Sperm To Power Up. Too Manly.

Perez, R. F. (2020, January 16). Ryan F Perez.

Pietrangelo, A. (2019a, June 4). Everything You Need to Know About Semen Retention.

Reid, R. C., Carpenter, B. N., & Fong, T. W. (2011). Neuroscience research fails to support claims that excessive pornography consumption causes brain damage. Surgical Neurology International, 2(1), 64. https://doi.org/10.4103/2152-7806.81427

Romano-Torres, M., Phillips-Farfán, B. V., Chavira, R., Rodríguez-Manzo, G., & Fernández-Guasti, A. (2007). Relationship between Sexual Satiety and Brain Androgen Receptors. Neuroendocrinology, 85(1), 16–26. https://doi.org/10.1159/000099250

Santos-Longhurst, A. (2020a, June 4). Are There Any Side Effects of Not Releasing Your Sperm (Ejaculating)?

Santos-Longhurst, A. (2020c, October 12). NoFap Benefits: Real or Overhyped?

Scaccia, A. (2019a, October 2). How to Increase Sexual Stamina: 45 Tips to Improve Strength, Endurance, and Technique.

Scaccia, A. (2019b, October 10). How to Practice Tantric Sex: 26

Tips for Masturbation and Partner Play.

Scaccia, A. (2019c, October 10). How to Practice Tantric Sex: 26 Tips for Masturbation and Partner Play.

Shambo, S. (2020, July 1). The Power of Semen Retention - Debunking The Prostate Cancer Myth. Tantric Academy. https://tantricacademy.com/semen-retention/

Sivananda. (2009, July 8). Ayurveda: Veerya, the Vital Fluid. Hindu Scriptures and Important Texts. https://gnosticteachings.org/scriptures/hindu/214-ayurveda-virya-the-vital-fluid.html

Sumit. (n.d.). 14 Serious Disadvantages of Masturbation-STOP IT RIGHT NOW! | Mr Mind Blowing. Retrieved October 31, 2020.

Sumit. (2020a, October 3). 17 Powerful Benefits Of Semen Retention (2020): A Warrior Strategy | Mr Mind Blowing.

Sumit. (2020b, October 3). 17 Powerful Benefits Of Semen Retention (2020): A Warrior Strategy | Mr Mind Blowing.

Sztajzel J, Périat M, Marti V, Krall P, Rutishauser W. Effect of sexual activity on cycle ergometer stress test parameters, on plasmatic testosterone levels and on concentration capacity. A study in high-level male athletes performed in the laboratory. J Sports Med Phys Fitness. 2000 Sep;40(3):233-9. PMID: 11125766.

Talib RA, Canguven O, Al-Rumaihi K, Al Ansari A, Alani M. The effect of fasting on erectile function and sexual desire on men in the month of Ramadan. Urology Journal. 2015 Apr;12(2):2099-2102.

REFERENCES

The Standard. (2013, October 27). How to take your mind off sex.

ThisAlpha.com. (2019, November 5). The Ultimate Guide To Semen Retention & Benefits.

Tyagi, V., Scordo, M., Yoon, R., Liporace, F.A., & Greene, L. (2017). Revisiting the role of testosterone: Are we missing something? Reviews in urology, 19 1, 16-24.

White, J. (n.d.). Semen Retention Benefits After 30 Days. Jonathan White Lifestyle.

Zayed, A. (2020, May 12). What Is Seminal Fluid Made of and Where Does It Come From?

www.ingramcontent.com/pod-product-compliance
Lightning Source LLC
Chambersburg PA
CBHW071520080526
44588CB00011B/1503